The Early Childhood Care and Education Workforce

CHALLENGES AND OPPORTUNITIES

A *Workshop* Report

Committee on Early Childhood Care and Education Workforce:
A Workshop

Board on Children, Youth, and Families

INSTITUTE OF MEDICINE *AND*
NATIONAL RESEARCH COUNCIL
OF THE NATIONAL ACADEMIES

THE NATIONAL ACADEMIES PRESS
Washington, D.C.
www.nap.edu

KH

THE NATIONAL ACADEMIES PRESS   500 Fifth Street, N.W.   Washington, DC 20001

NOTICE: The project that is the subject of this report was approved by the Governing Board of the National Research Council, whose members are drawn from the councils of the National Academy of Sciences, the National Academy of Engineering, and the Institute of Medicine.

This study was supported by Contract No. HHSP23337014T between the National Academy of Sciences and the U.S. Department of Health and Human Services. Any opinions, findings, conclusions, or recommendations expressed in this publication are those of the author(s) and do not necessarily reflect the view of the organizations or agencies that provided support for this project.

International Standard Book Number-13:   978-0-309-21934-1
International Standard Book Number-10:   0-309-21934-5

Additional copies of this report are available from The National Academies Press, 500 Fifth Street, N.W., Lockbox 285, Washington, DC 20055; (800) 624-6242 or (202) 334-3313 (in the Washington metropolitan area); Internet, http://www.nap.edu.

For more information about the Institute of Medicine, visit the IOM home page at: **www.iom.edu.**

The serpent has been a symbol of long life, healing, and knowledge among almost all cultures and religions since the beginning of recorded history. The serpent adopted as a logotype by the Institute of Medicine is a relief carving from ancient Greece, now held by the Staatliche Museen in Berlin.

Suggested citation: IOM (Institute of Medicine) and NRC (National Research Council). 2012. *The early childhood care and education workforce: Challenges and opportunities: A workshop report.* Washington, DC: The National Academies Press.

5/1/13

ERRATA

On page 1, the following text is a correction to the fourth sentence of the second paragraph:

Current estimates indicate that more than half of the 25.5 million U.S. children under age 6 spend time in the regular care of someone other than a parent in a typical week (Federal Interagency Forum on Child and Family Statistics, 2011; Iruka and Carver, 2006).

On page 93, the reference for Guzman et al., 2009, was deleted and the following reference was added:

Federal Interagency Forum on Child and Family Statistics. 2011. *America's children: Key national indicators of well-being, 2011.* Washington, DC: U.S. Government Printing Office. http:// www.childstats.gov/pdf/ac2011/ac_11.pdf (accessed February 16, 2012).

On page 94, the following reference was added:

Iruka, I. U., and P. R. Carver. 2006. *Initial results from the 2005 NHES Early Childhood Program Participation Survey (NCES 2006-075).* U.S. Department of Education. Washington, DC: National Center for Education Statistics. http://nces.ed.gov/ pubs2006/2006075.pdf (accessed February 16, 2012).

The addition of the reference on page 94 caused text to shift on pages 94-97.

The Early Childhood Care and Education Workforce: Challenges and Opportunities: A Workshop Report
The National Academies Press, Washington, DC
2012
ISBN-13: 978-0-309-21934-1
ISBN-10: 0-309-21934-5

THE NATIONAL ACADEMIES
Advisers to the Nation on Science, Engineering, and Medicine

The **National Academy of Sciences** is a private, nonprofit, self-perpetuating society of distinguished scholars engaged in scientific and engineering research, dedicated to the furtherance of science and technology and to their use for the general welfare. Upon the authority of the charter granted to it by the Congress in 1863, the Academy has a mandate that requires it to advise the federal government on scientific and technical matters. Dr. Ralph J. Cicerone is president of the National Academy of Sciences.

The **National Academy of Engineering** was established in 1964, under the charter of the National Academy of Sciences, as a parallel organization of outstanding engineers. It is autonomous in its administration and in the selection of its members, sharing with the National Academy of Sciences the responsibility for advising the federal government. The National Academy of Engineering also sponsors engineering programs aimed at meeting national needs, encourages education and research, and recognizes the superior achievements of engineers. Dr. Charles M. Vest is president of the National Academy of Engineering.

The **Institute of Medicine** was established in 1970 by the National Academy of Sciences to secure the services of eminent members of appropriate professions in the examination of policy matters pertaining to the health of the public. The Institute acts under the responsibility given to the National Academy of Sciences by its congressional charter to be an adviser to the federal government and, upon its own initiative, to identify issues of medical care, research, and education. Dr. Harvey V. Fineberg is president of the Institute of Medicine.

The **National Research Council** was organized by the National Academy of Sciences in 1916 to associate the broad community of science and technology with the Academy's purposes of furthering knowledge and advising the federal government. Functioning in accordance with general policies determined by the Academy, the Council has become the principal operating agency of both the National Academy of Sciences and the National Academy of Engineering in providing services to the government, the public, and the scientific and engineering communities. The Council is administered jointly by both Academies and the Institute of Medicine. Dr. Ralph J. Cicerone and Dr. Charles M. Vest are chair and vice chair, respectively, of the National Research Council.

www.national-academies.org

COMMITTEE ON EARLY CHILDHOOD CARE AND EDUCATION WORKFORCE: A WORKSHOP

ALETHA C. HUSTON (*Chair*), Priscilla Pond Flawn Regents Professor of Child Development, Human Development and Family Sciences, The University of Texas at Austin

DAVID M. BLAU, SBS Distinguished Professor of Economics, The Ohio State University, Columbus

RICHARD N. BRANDON, Principal, RNB Consulting, Seattle, WA

JEANNE BROOKS-GUNN, Virginia and Leonard Marx Professor of Child Development and Education, Teachers College, Columbia University, New York

VIRGINIA BUYSSE, Senior Scientist, Frank Porter Graham Child Development Institute, The University of North Carolina at Chapel Hill

DEBORAH J. CASSIDY, Director, North Carolina Division of Child Development, North Carolina Department of Health and Human Services, Raleigh, NC

CATHERINE DOWER, Associate Director, Research, Center for the Health Professions, University of California, San Francisco

YOLANDA GARCIA, Director, West Ed E3 Institute-Excellence in Early Education, San Jose, CA

SHARON LYNN KAGAN, Professor of Early Childhood and Family Policy, Columbia University, Teachers College, New York

ROBERT G. LYNCH, Professor of Economics, Chair, Department of Economics, Washington College, Chestertown, MD

DIXIE SOMMERS, Assistant Commissioner, Occupational Statistics and Employment Projections, Bureau of Labor Statistics, U.S. Department of Labor, Washington, DC

MARCY WHITEBOOK, Director and Senior Researcher, Center for the Study of Child Care Employment, University of California, Berkeley

Study Staff

HOLLY RHODES, *Study Director*
ALEXANDRA BEATTY, *Senior Program Officer*
REINE Y. HOMAWOO, *Senior Program Assistant*
ROSEMARY CHALK, *Board Director*
WENDY KEENAN, *Program Associate*
JULIENNE PALBUSA, *Research Assistant*

Reviewers

This report has been reviewed in draft form by individuals chosen for their diverse perspectives and technical expertise, in accordance with procedures approved by the National Research Council's Report Review Committee. The purpose of this independent review is to provide candid and critical comments that will assist the institution in making its published report as sound as possible and to ensure that the report meets institutional standards for objectivity, evidence, and responsiveness to the study charge. The review comments and draft manuscript remain confidential to protect the integrity of the process. We wish to thank the following individuals for their review of this report:

Harriet Dichter, First Five Years Fund
Eugene Garcia, Arizona State University
Robert Pianta, University of Virginia

Although the reviewers listed above have provided many constructive comments and suggestions, they were not asked to endorse the final draft of the report before its release. The review of this report was overseen by **Caswell A. Evans** of the University of Illinois at Chicago. Appointed by the National Research Council and Institute of Medicine, he was responsible for making certain that an independent examination of this report was carried out in accordance with institutional procedures and that all review comments were carefully considered. Responsibility for the final content of this report rests entirely with the authors and the institution.

Preface

More than 30 years ago, *Children at the Center* (Ruopp and Irwin, 1979) called attention to the important role of teachers and caregivers who were serving an increasing percentage of young children. A decade later the National Child Care Staffing Study (Whitebook et al., 1990) brought the issues of teacher education and training, turnover, and wages to the forefront of national discussion and established their link to the quality of caregiving. Over the years, such major studies as the Cost, Quality, and Child Outcomes Study (Helburn, 1995) and the National Institute of Child Health and Human Development Study of Early Child Care (NICHD, 2002) firmly established the importance of quality care to the well-being of children and their later success. The long-term follow-up of the Perry Preschool (Schweinhart et al., 1993) and Abecedarian programs (Campbell and Ramey, 1995) documented the economic benefits to investing in early childhood programs. Earlier reports from the National Research Council (NRC) and the Institute of Medicine (IOM), such as *Who Cares for America's Children?* (NRC, 1990), *From Neurons to Neighborhoods* (NRC and IOM, 2000), and *Eager to Learn* (NRC, 2001), synthesized the child development research, showing the critical nature of the birth-to-age-5 period of life for later success, the importance of quality experiences for children, and the central role of teachers and caregivers in early childhood care and education settings.

The research picture is clear—quality of care and education matters to the lives of young children, and teachers and caregivers are central to providing that quality. Fittingly, initiatives at the state and federal levels have sought to bolster the skills and knowledge of the workforce, to tie their educational attainment to higher pay, and to reduce teacher turnover. Yet, the problems identified more than 30 years ago—inadequate training and education, low wages, and high turnover—are still vexing today (Herzenberg et al., 2005; Kagan et al., 2008; Whitebook, 2003; Whitebook et al., 2001). To tackle these issues, policy makers need a complete picture of teachers and caregivers—their professional preparation, working conditions, compensation, training, and qualifications. Knowing how many teachers and caregivers are in the workforce and how economic forces affect it is the starting point for making decisions about the most cost-effective ways to build the profession of early childhood care and education (ECCE) in ways that ultimately benefit children and families. Although such information appears to be straightforward, in practice painting a comprehensive picture of the ECCE workforce is quite complex. Detailed data are available for segments of the workforce such as state prekindergarten programs and Head Start, but are much sparser for family, home-based, and relative child care. The lack of consensus on a definition of the ECCE workforce poses a fundamental challenge.

The Committee on Early Childhood Care and Education Workforce was asked to plan a workshop sponsored by the Board on Children, Youth, and Families of the IOM and NRC, with support from the Administration for Children and Families (ACF) in the U.S. Department of Health and Human Services to address this challenge. This effort was encouraged by the leadership of Joan Lombardi, deputy assistant secretary and interdepartmental liaison for early childhood development at ACF, who sought to bring needed attention to the ECCE workforce. Our committee's primary charge was to plan a workshop that would provide an adequate description of the workforce and to outline the parameters that define the population.

Thus, we organized the workshop around three key areas: (1) defining and describing the ECCE workforce; (2) exploring characteristics of the ECCE workforce that impact children; and (3) describing the context that shapes the workforce and how to build the profession of early childhood care and education. This report summarizes the presentations and discussions from the workshop. As a workshop report, this report does not reflect the conclusions or judgments of the committee, but rather describes the research and perspectives that were presented. The report also includes two commissioned papers. The first presents a description of the ECCE workforce based on a review of federal data sources and 50 research studies. This paper also includes detailed descriptions of all of the reviewed studies. The second paper offers a detailed description of relevant federal data sources, the elements they include, their structure, and their benefits and drawbacks for obtaining data on the ECCE workforce.

The committee would like to thank the study director for this project, Holly Rhodes, for overseeing the project from its inception; Alexandra Beatty for providing an initial draft of the report from which the report was developed; and Reine Homawoo for excellent logistical and project support. We also gratefully acknowledge the contributions of report editor, Laura Penny and report review officer, Elisabeth Reese. Finally, the committee extends sincere thanks to Joan Lombardi and T'Pring Westbrook, and their colleagues at the Administration for Children and Families for their support.

Aletha C. Huston, *Chair*
Committee on Early Childhood
Care and Education Workforce:
A Workshop

Contents

1

Introduction

Early childhood is a period of enormous growth and development. Children are developing more rapidly during the period from birth to age 5 than at any other time in their lives, shaped in large part by their experiences in the world. These early years of development are critical for providing a firm foundation in cognitive, language, and motor development, as well as social, emotional, regulatory, and moral development (NRC and IOM, 2000). Stimulating, nurturing, and stable relationships with parents and other caregivers are of prime importance to children's healthy development, and the absence of these factors can compromise children's development.

The individuals who comprise the early childhood care and education (ECCE) workforce are important providers of these early experiences. They form meaningful bonds with the children in their care, and their interactions, behaviors, and teaching practices all influence children's development, as well as their later school readiness (NRC, 2001; Peisner-Feinberg et al., 2001; Pianta and Stuhlman, 2004). Moreover, they are affecting the development of an increasing proportion of U.S. children. Current estimates indicate that more than half of the 12 million U.S. children under age 6 spend time in the regular care of someone other than a parent in a typical week, and 85 percent by the time they reach kindergarten (Guzman et al., 2009). These arrangements can include center-based child care, preschool, family child care centers, or informal care arrangements with friends, family, and neighbors, both paid and unpaid.

The term "early childhood care and education" is inclusive of all these arrangements.

Policy-maker and public perception of ECCE is frequently at odds with the weighty responsibilities of this workforce, who influence so many facets of children's development both in the short and long terms (Karoly et al., 2005). As the authors of *From Neurons to Neighborhoods* concluded:

> The time is long overdue for society to recognize the significance of out-of-home relationships for young children, to esteem those who care for them when their parents are not available, and to compensate them adequately as a means of supporting stability, and quality in these relationships for all children, regardless of their families' income and irrespective of their developmental needs. (NRC and IOM, 2000, p. 7)

Ten years since the publication of that report, most teachers and caregivers continue to receive low wages and to have low status, and are often described as "babysitters" or as "watching" children. Teachers in publicly funded preschool settings have fared somewhat better, but even these positions are viewed as low-status roles compared with elementary and secondary educators. The results of these circumstances include high turnover and few career opportunities in the field (Kagan et al., 2008).

The primary purpose of the early care or educational setting plays a role in shaping the perceptions and expectations for the workforce. Bellm and Whitebook (2006) describe two types of ECCE services—those with an educational focus and those whose primary function is to provide a safe setting that meets the basic needs of children of working parents. These purposes shape the terminology that describes the workforce (e.g., teachers versus caregivers), as well as policies and regulations at the local, state, and federal levels (Bellm and Whitebook, 2006).

Real differences between settings on degree of focus on educational goals relative to caring for children's basic needs exist. However, opportunities to nurture healthy development and early learning occur in all of these settings, and some argue that children in all settings should experience effective practices regardless of the primary purpose of the care arrangement (NAEYC, 2009). Some have also argued that a workforce that can implement research-based practices is essential, not only because these high-quality experiences are beneficial to children, but also more importantly because the low-quality experiences that are so prevalent actually can harm children's development and contribute to a widening achievement gap prior to kindergarten (Pianta et al., 2009).

These practices include providing a rich environment and nurturing care, teaching in an intentional manner, and making effective decisions in creative and appropriate ways (Hamre and Pianta, 2005; NAEYC, 2009;

Pianta et al., 2008). Ideally, this approach involves implementing curriculums, individually tailoring activities, and assessing progress, while responding flexibly to the varied personalities and basic care needs of the children and families they serve, all tasks that demand knowledge, skills, and flexibility. Adding to these demands are the greater numbers of children in poverty and children who are English-language learners, many of whom are from immigrant families (Garcia and Frede, 2010; Suárez-Orozco and Suárez-Orozco, 2001). These particular groups of children most frequently need these high-quality experiences and yet have limited access to them (NRC, 2001).

Studies have examined particular segments of the workforce (e.g., Head Start or state prekindergarten programs), but few data exist about this workforce as a whole to help policy makers develop strategies for improving early childhood care and education, or to evaluate the effectiveness of those policies (Brandon and Martinez-Beck, 2006). The available data indicate that the workforce is largely female and poorly compensated (see Chapter 2; Kagan et al., 2008); however, they vary widely in many other ways shaped by contextual factors at various levels. Working conditions, compensation, professional development opportunities, incentives and systems of recognition, and administrative support, as well as policies at the federal, state, and local levels, constitute the context that shape how this vital workforce functions.

ABOUT THE WORKSHOP AND THIS REPORT

Recognition of the critical importance of the ECCE workforce and the lack of attention that has been paid to it provided the impetus for a workshop conducted in Washington, DC, in March 2011 by the Board on Children, Youth, and Families of the Institute of Medicine and National Research Council, with the support of the Administration for Children and Families of the U.S. Department of Health and Human Services. Over a day and a half, the workshop consisted of invited presentations, as well as discussion periods with discussant panels and workshop participants. More than 70 participants attended the workshop, in addition to planning committee members and invited speakers. Participants included researchers, policy analysts, association representatives, university faculty and administrators, leaders of state early childhood programs, administrators of ECCE programs, individuals involved with professional development, and federal staff from various agencies.

The primary purpose of the workshop was to provide an adequate description of the ECCE workforce, outlining the parameters that define that population. The planning committee interpreted this charge as encompassing three areas of examination: (1) defining and describing the nature of the current ECCE workforce; (2) examining the characteristics of the workforce that affect the development of children; and (3) describing the context of the workforce and how best to build the ECCE profession in ways that promote program quality and effective child outcomes, while supporting the essential individuals who provide care and education.

The workshop presentations and discussions are described in this report. Chapter 2 focuses on ways to define, quantify, and describe the early childhood care and education workforce, and Chapter 3 discusses some of the economic and policy issues that affect it. Chapter 4 examines the effects that the characteristics of this workforce may have on children and their families, and Chapter 5 presents prospects for understanding the challenges that face the workforce and strategies for building the workforce and the profession. The final chapter summarizes the key themes that emerged from the presentations and discussions. The agenda, a list of workshop participants, and materials commissioned for the workshop are included as appendixes. These materials include two papers that summarize a review of the data on the ECCE workforce and provide relevant background information on selected federal workforce data systems. The presentations and other materials from the workshop may be found on the National Academies website at http://www.bocyf.org/early_childcare_workforce_workshop.html. This workshop report[1] was prepared through collaboration among the study staff and the workshop planning committee.

---

[1] The report summarizes the views expressed by workshop participants. Although the committee is responsible for the overall quality and accuracy of the report as a record of what transpired at the workshop, the views contained in the report are not necessarily those of the committee.

2

Defining and Describing the Workforce

Understanding the characteristics and roles of the early childhood care and education (ECCE) workforce is not a straightforward task. Even counting the number of workers engaged in the care and education of young children raises questions—about whom to include and how to categorize the nature of their work, for example.

The committee was charged to plan a workshop that would yield a description of the early childhood workforce and outline the parameters that define it. However, the field currently lacks a clear conceptual definition and comprehensive data on the ECCE workforce on which presentations of existing data could be based. Thus, Richard Brandon, principal at RNB Consulting, in collaboration with several colleagues,[1] developed an initial conceptual definition as a starting point for discussion of key issues in defining and describing the ECCE workforce (see Appendix B). In addition, the planning committee commissioned Michelle Maroto at the University of Washington to work with Brandon to review existing federal data sources and published research studies and to compile currently available descriptive data on the ECCE workforce. Brandon presented both the conceptual definition and descriptive data on the ECCE workforce at the workshop. Additional presentations focused on the nature of federal workforce data systems, an innovative state model for improving ECCE workforce data systems, and lessons learned from K–12 federal data systems.

---

[1] David Blau, Sharon Lynn Kagan, Dixie Sommers, and Marcy Whitebook.

DEFINING THE WORKFORCE—A FRESH LOOK

The ECCE workforce is exceptionally varied, a fact that reflects the varying purposes for which care and education are provided and the varying expectations of those who fund and oversee it. The workforce is composed of individuals with little or no training who provide mainly custodial care without attention to educational goals at one end of the spectrum, to individuals with specialized postgraduate degrees providing carefully planned educational experiences at the other, with many others in between. At its most basic level, caregiving can involve caring or providing for a child's safety, meeting basic needs around feeding, diapering, or toileting, and assisting with dressing, bathing, and sleep routines. At its most complex, teaching can involve carefully implementing research-based curriculums, individualizing care and instruction, and addressing the full range of developmental domains (e.g., cognitive, language, social–emotional, fine and gross motor, executive functioning) in groups and one-on-one activities.

Terminology can be problematic with such a wide spectrum of work represented, even among the members of the workforce themselves. For example, those working in settings whose primary purpose is educational are often referred to as teachers. The terms "caregiver," "child care worker," or "child care provider" are more often associated with settings whose primary purpose is enabling parents to work. Those who provide child care, particularly through informal friend, family, or neighbor relationships, may not see themselves as having any particular job title as either caregivers or teachers. This makes selecting an appropriate term for the full range of members of the ECCE workforce challenging. This report uses the terms, "ECCE workforce" or "caregivers and teachers" as a means for being inclusive. The terms "workforce" or "workers" refer to anyone who works for pay. Using these definitions, the planning committee focused the workshop primarily on those who are paid for providing early care and education.

The full range of care and education can be offered in a variety of settings (e.g., private homes, centers, elementary schools, workplaces, or houses of worship), funded by numerous sources (e.g., parent tuition, child care subsidies, state funds, and federal dollars), and licensed or unlicensed. Many children are cared for by family, friends, and neighbors, both paid and unpaid. Despite these differences in location, funding, or licensed status, the primary purpose of the setting (i.e., providing education or enabling a parent to work) may be the most important dimension on which settings differ, along with how well that purpose is implemented (Pianta et al., 2009). Settings established for these differing purposes may be governed by differing sets of rules and expectations, which can affect variation in workforce characteristics. The teachers and caregivers within these settings are nearly all women receiving low pay for their work, but they are also diverse in many respects (e.g., demographic characteristics qualifications, knowledge, beliefs, and attitudes). Whatever their characteristics and qualifications, these teachers and caregivers have a profound impact on the lives of children and families (see Chapter 4). Therefore, clearly defining, describing, and monitoring this workforce over time is important.

Brandon presented selection criteria that could be used to develop shared definitions of terms and categories, which might then support efforts to achieve greater consistency and improve research and policy making. The conceptual definition Brandon presented focused on children from birth to age 5, and used criteria consistent with the distinctions applied by the Bureau of Labor Statistics (BLS) between *occupations* (roles and functions) and *sectors* of the economy or *industries* (the organizations or establishments that provided particular services). (These are discussed further below.) These distinctions are important, he explained, because consistent definitions will allow researchers to build on the considerable investment that has already been made in federal data systems, rather than developing new, separate definitions for the early childhood sector. Consistency will also support comparisons of the ECCE workforce to workers in other economic sectors, as well as analyses of their key features. Moreover, Brandon pointed out, distinguishing and cross-tabulating occupations by sectors provides opportunities for analyses that can lead to improvements in recruitment, training, and professional development.

Despite the potential benefits of consistency, Brandon enumerated a number of concerns with the existing federal definitions of the early childhood workforce. For example, the existing federal data system groups together those who work with young children and those who work with school-aged children (with some exceptions described later in this chapter). This is a problem because "the duties are very different for dealing with young children and school-aged children," Brandon observed. Thus, he hoped to provide points to be considered in future revisions to the federal definitions that would make them more accurate and useful. Brandon and his colleagues developed a definition that includes three primary components: *occupation, sector,* and *enterprise*. Figure 2-1 provides a visual representation of these components.

A first step was to define the **occupation** clearly. All federal agencies, including the BLS and the Census Bureau, use the Standard Occupational Classification (SOC) to identify distinct occupations based on the nature of the work performed. According to the Classification Principles and Coding Guidelines of the *2010 Standard Occupational Classification Manual (SOC Manual)*, "the SOC covers all occupations in which work is performed for pay or profit" (OMB, 2010, p. 1). Thus, in the case of early

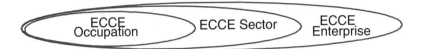

FIGURE 2-1 Components of the early childhood care and education (ECCE) workforce.
SOURCE: Brandon, 2011.

childhood workers, Brandon and his colleagues identified two criteria for inclusion: (1) the work involves direct care for or education of infants and children from birth through age 5,[2] and (2) the worker is paid for this work. These criteria were designed to distinguish early childhood workers from others who work with children, such as social workers, family counselors, or nurses and pediatricians. Teachers and child care workers would be included, as would proprietors or directors of child care centers, specialists, and family support workers or home visitors, as long as they work directly with children, rather than only with adults.

This definition includes family members, friends, and neighbors who provide care, as long as they are paid. Brandon expressed the view that this definition is "radically broader than anything in [the current] federal data systems." Individuals who provide unpaid care or instruction would not be included. Brandon acknowledged that these unpaid caregivers are a sizeable and important group and pose a challenge for the field to consider. He suggested that this group should be the subject of future analyses. He noted that the Census Bureau defines a worker who is paid for at least 1 hour of work during the week in which data were collected as a member of an occupation, and that "we have to think both about what makes sense within the field and what makes it possible to compare early care and education workers to other workers."

To define the ECCE **sector**, Brandon and his colleagues considered the employers of individuals in the occupation. The North American Industry Classification System (NAICS) maintained by the Office of Management and Budget (OMB) classifies businesses by the type of product produced or service provided. They applied this approach to the ECCE workforce. Thus, the ECCE *sector* includes those people in the *occupation* whose paid work involves direct instruction or care of young children, as well as others who work for establishments that provide such care, such as non-

---

[2] During discussion, Brandon clarified that he selected "care *or* education to be maximally inclusive of all paid ECCE workers." A number of participants indicated that they preferred the term "care *and* education."

teaching directors or supervisors, trainers, or those involved in administrative, transportation, food service, or janitorial services.

Brandon also described a broader category, the **enterprise**, which includes all individuals involved in the ECCE sector as well as others whose paid work has a direct effect on caregiving or educational practice, such as professional development providers, mentors, and coaches employed by entities outside of the sector; those employed by states or local jurisdictions to provide referrals or resources or run licensure programs; and university faculty who teach prospective teachers. The enterprise does not have a defined counterpart within the federal classification systems, but Brandon and his colleagues considered it important to represent the contributions of this broader group. This category would also include family support workers or home visitors who work primarily with parents and not with children because their work may influence children or child care workers, Brandon noted. It would not include advocates or policy makers who may nevertheless have an influence on the nature of early childhood programs.

Workshop participants had many comments and questions about these conceptual definitions. Some cautioned that the definition of the occupation might be too exclusive, for example, because it excludes home visitors or special educators, whose primary functions may be working with parents or other teachers as a means of affecting child development. One noted that professional societies have "worked hard to make sure that ... everybody in the building ... understands that they contribute to the growth and development of children." Participants also reinforced the point that lack of data on the contribution of unpaid workers is a significant challenge to policy makers.

Another cautioned against being too inclusive, however, arguing that overly broad classification criteria will make it difficult to evaluate the impact of the workforce on the quality of care and education, as well as on child development. Although it is important to recognize the range of individual contributions, one participant suggested that more rigor is necessary to achieve consistency in measurement. Another participant agreed, noting that including speech–language pathologists or others who belong to another well-defined profession may add an unnecessary complication. More than one participant raised the challenges of crafting a definition that fit the roles of those working with children with special needs. For example, teachers, caregivers, and specialists may share similar responsibilities for working directly with these children. This blurring of roles can make distinguishing one occupation from another difficult.

Several participants raised concerns regarding the terminology used in the definitions, noting, for example, that it is important to view the work as a combination of care *and* instruction, rather than care *or* instruction.

All providers should be expected to offer "direct support for development and learning," one observed. Yet others questioned the word "instruction," suggesting that "education" or "intentionality" may be more appropriate terms for work with very young children and infants. Participants' comments indicated that the conceptual definition of the ECCE workforce has practical implications for data collecting and reporting, as well as policy implications for how the field itself and others view it. Several participants noted that a desire for consistency with federal data systems could be difficult to reconcile with the need to capture unique aspects of ECCE, including the diverse work settings, team-based approaches, and progressive roles. Committee members encouraged participants to continue sharing their ideas for further honing a workable conceptual definition of the ECCE workforce that would serve both data and policy goals.

THE FEDERAL STATISTICAL SYSTEM

Data collected by the federal government is the source of most of the current national information about the ECCE workforce. Understanding these federal data systems is needed as ECCE considers how to define its occupational borders in ways that promote accuracy and comparability with other occupations. Dixie Sommers, assistant commissioner, BLS, U.S. Department of Labor, provided an overview of the type of information that is collected and how the system is structured.

The three primary sources of federal data on the ECCE workforce are: (1) the BLS, (2) the Census Bureau (within the U.S. Department of Commerce), and (3) the National Center for Education Statistics (NCES) (within the U.S. Department of Education). The federal statistical system is decentralized, Sommers explained, with individual federal statistical agencies responsible for data collection that pertains to their missions. The OMB oversees data collection standards through its Office of Information and Regulatory Affairs. This office sets policies—for example, to protect the privacy of respondents or standardize classifications of information—and also coordinates data collection to prevent redundancy across agencies.

The purpose of standardizing classifications is to ensure that data collected across agencies can be compared, Sommers explained. Interagency committees made up of federal experts in statistics and in the relevant fields or occupational areas make recommendations about data collection based on research and public comment, and the OMB establishes and revises the standards in response to these recommendations. The classification systems cover four broad areas: industries, occupations, metropolitan areas, and race/ethnicity categories. As noted above, NAICS classifies businesses by type of product produced or service provided, and includes child care or instructional providers. However, it does not distinguish providers by the ages of the children served or identify those who are part of an establishment that has another primary purpose (e.g., a child care center in an elementary school because the child care center is not a stand-alone business). Table 2-1 illustrates how the NAICS defines the three industries that are most relevant to ECCE: elementary and secondary schools, child day-care services, and private households (in which paid child care is provided).

The SOC classifies jobs and workers according to the nature of the tasks and functions performed, and sometimes the qualifications associated with them. Classification principles and coding guidelines are used to guide decisions to add new occupations or change existing ones, Sommers explained. For example, principles guide the classification of managers and supervisors and how to determine whether a particular type of work constitutes a new occupation. Box 2-1 presents the definitions of two ECCE occupations from the *SOC Manual* (OMB, 2010). The 2010 edition of the *SOC Manual* included a few changes in the early childhood context, such as distinguishing special education preschool teachers from special education kindergarten teachers.

Sommers noted a few problems with the existing federal definitions in comparison with the conceptual definition of the ECCE workforce pre-

TABLE 2-1 Definitions Used in the North American Industry Classification System

Code and Title	Definition
611110 Elementary and Secondary Schools	Establishments primarily engaged in furnishing academic courses and associated course work that comprise a basic preparatory education. A basic preparatory education ordinarily constitutes kindergarten through 12th grade. This industry includes school boards and school districts.
624410 Child Day Care Services	Establishments primarily engaged in providing day care of infants or children. These establishments generally care for preschool children, but may care for older children when they are not in school and may also offer prekindergarten educational programs.
814110 Private Households	Private households primarily engaged in employing workers on or about the premises in activities primarily concerned with the operation of the household. These private households may employ individuals, such as cooks, maids, nannies, butlers, and outside workers, such as gardeners, caretakers, and other maintenance workers.

SOURCE: Sommers, 2011. Based on OMB, 2007.

BOX 2-1
Definitions from the
***2010 Standard Occupational Classification Manual* (OMB, 2010)**

Preschool Teachers, Except Special Education (code 25-2011)
Instruct preschool children in activities designed to promote social, physical, and intellectual growth needed for primary school in preschool, day care center, or other child development facility. Substitute teachers are included in "Teachers and Instructors, All Other" (25-3099). May be required to hold state certification. Excludes "Childcare Workers" (39-9011) and "Special Education Teachers" (25-2050).

Childcare Workers (code 39-9011)
Attend to children at schools, businesses, private households, and child care institutions. Perform a variety of tasks, such as dressing, feeding, bathing, and overseeing play. Excludes "Preschool Teachers, Except Special Education" (25-2011) and "Teacher Assistants" (25-9041).

SOURCE: OMB, 2010.

sented earlier. They do not consistently distinguish workers who care for or educate children from birth through age 5 from those who work with school-aged children. Furthermore, researchers in the field indicate that the definitions of child care workers and preschool teachers do not reflect the reality of their work, especially the overlap in their respective roles.

Sommers provided a list of federal data sources that provide information relevant to the early childhood sector. Table 2-2 includes only the data sources produced by the BLS and the Census Bureau. She pointed out different methods of collecting information, each of which has strengths and weaknesses, in terms of the type of information collected, the level of detail possible, and other factors. For example, household surveys such as the Current Population Survey and the American Community Survey provide a broad look at the entire paid labor force, including those who are self-employed and those who are "unpaid family workers," but they may not provide the desired level of detail about particular occupations or industries. The BLS' business establishment survey, the Occupational Employment Statistics (OES) survey, yields more detail about occupations than the household surveys do. In addition, this survey's large sample size yields considerable detail by industry and geographic region. These establishments are sampled from a business list that is based on administrative data (mainly unemployment insurance tax reports). The survey does not collect demographic information, however.

Further information on these federal data systems may be found in a

TABLE 2-2 Standard Federal Data Sources

Source	Employment by Industry	Employment by Occupation	Includes Self-Employed	Geographic Detail	Demographic Characteristics
		Census Bureau, Household Surveys			
Current Population Survey (CPS)	Less than full detail	Less than full detail	Yes	State, MSA	Yes
American Community Survey (ACS)	Less than full detail	Less than full detail	Yes	Small area detail	Yes
		Bureau of Labor Statistics, Establishment Surveys			
Current Employment Statistics (CES)	Significant detail	No	No	State, MSA	No
Occupational Employment Statistics (OES)	4-digit NAICS	Nearly full detail	No	State, MSA, non-metro areas	No
		Bureau of Labor Statistics, Administrative Data			
Quarterly Census of Employment and Wages (QCEW)	Full NAICS detail	No	No	State, county	No

NOTE: MSA: Metropolitan Statistical Area; NAICS: North American Industry Classification System.
SOURCE: Sommers, 2011.

paper Sommers prepared for this workshop that is included in Appendix B. This detailed report: (1) describes the SOC and the NAICS in detail; (2) discusses issues specific to ECCE related to these systems; and (3) profiles relevant BLS and Census data sources, including key meta-data and the advantages and limitations of each source for understanding the ECCE workforce.

DESCRIBING THE WORKFORCE

In planning the workshop, the planning committee noted both that the federal data sources do not correspond completely to the reality of the jobs early childhood workers do, and that these data systems are not designed to capture all of the types of information that would be useful to have about this workforce. Therefore, they commissioned Michelle Maroto, who collaborated with Richard Brandon to review available descriptive data and to compile a portrait of the ECCE workforce (see Appendix B for the complete review). Also included in Appendix B with this descriptive summary of findings is a complete list and bulleted description of each study reviewed, including the study title, researching organization, purpose, design, sample, methods, limitations, and associated references for each study reviewed. In addition, spreadsheets of the data gathered to compile the description of the workforce were prepared and will be made available on the Institute of Medicine (IOM) project website.

The authors selected 50 studies for review, assigning greater weight to those that were nationally representative and included the most different types of child care settings. The studies they included covered all types of teachers and caregivers who work with children from birth to age 5 (except those who are unpaid friends, family members, or neighbors). In many cases, preschool teacher data also included data about kindergarten teachers because data from the Census Bureau do not distinguish between these two types of teachers.[3] Brandon summarized their findings at the workshop.

To complement the review of federal data sources and existing research studies, Brandon reported on his recent work to identify the number of ECCE workers in the workforce (Brandon et al., 2011). This estimate of the size of the workforce was based on data from the National Household Education Survey Early Childhood Supplement, 2005, which includes parent reports about where their children spend time and the ratio of children to adults in child care settings. From these data and some

---

[3] Tabulations of previously unpublished data from Census and BLS sources regarding worker characteristics and benefits are provided in the accompanying background paper, Appendix B.

statistical adjustments, the authors calculated the number of individuals required to provide the care. This method made it possible to break the numbers down by the ages of the children: approximately one-fourth of the paid workers are caring for infants, one-third for toddlers, and nearly half for children ages 3 to 5 (see Appendix B for further details; the full analysis is published in Brandon et al., 2011). Using these methods, Brandon reported an estimate of approximately 2.2 million individuals who are paid members of the ECCE workforce. These workers make up a significant proportion (approximately 30 percent) of the overall instructional workforce in the United States, which includes those engaged in teaching at the early education, elementary, secondary, and postsecondary levels (Brandon et al., 2011). An additional 3.2 million individuals provide non-parental care without being paid. Figure 2-2 shows how these workers are distributed among different types of settings.

Using the review that he and Maroto completed, Brandon described the demographic characteristics of the paid ECCE workforce. He noted that the Census Bureau provides the most current nationally representative data on the workforce, but does not distinguish among those who work in different types of settings (child care, preschool, or elementary school settings; licensed versus unlicensed), or between preschool from kindergarten teachers. One of the primary concerns about these data, he noted, is that they include public school kindergarten teachers. Teachers in K–12 schools often have to meet minimum qualifications that most workers in other early childhood settings are not required to meet. There-

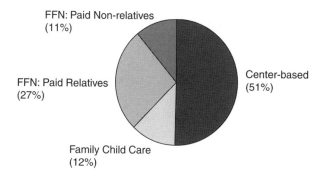

FIGURE 2-2 The paid early childhood care and education (ECCE) workforce by type of worker, 2005.
NOTE: FFN = Friends, Family, and Neighbors.
SOURCE: Brandon et al., 2011.

fore, Brandon focused on characteristics "where there is no particular reason to assume that characteristics of people caring for young children are substantially different from those who include school-aged children" for his presentation.

These data indicate that the median age for these workers is 39 to 47, that 90 to 98 percent of them are female, and that 75 to 80 percent of teachers and 81 to 85 percent of directors are non-Hispanic whites. Of the total population, 48 percent are married, 33 percent never married, and 18 percent were formerly married. Sixty-eight percent have children living at home.

Brandon described a serious wage penalty for those who work in the early childhood sector: women working in early child care (other than preschool) earn 31 percent less than women with similar qualifications working in other occupations[4] (Brandon et al., 2011). These workers' annual earnings range from approximately $31,000 for preschool and kindergarten teachers, $21,000 for assistant teachers, to approximately $18,000 for other child care workers. Paid family child care workers earn an average of about $14,000 per year. Four to 5 percent of teachers have a second job, and 3 percent of family child care workers do. Annual median household incomes (in 2010 dollars) are about $40,000 for child care workers (based on data from the Cost, Quality and Child Outcomes Study; Helburn, 1995) and about $68,000 for prekindergarten teachers (National Prekindergarten Study; Gilliam and Marchesseault, 2005), as compared with the current approximate $60,000 median for all households.[5]

Brandon described the qualifications of this workforce, noting that, "we see across the different categories of workers a very great range of educational background." He reported that among child care workers, 7 to 12 percent have an associate's degree (A.A.), 13 to 21 percent have a bachelor's degree (B.A.), and 2 to 4 percent have a master's degree (M.A.) or professional degree. Twenty-four to 25 percent of preschool teachers have gone beyond the B.A., and just 2 to 4 percent of family child care workers have done so. Estimates of how many preschool teachers with a Child Development Associate (CDA) credential range from 23 to 76 percent. Twenty-nine to 57 percent of preschool teachers have state certification, and 34 to 39 percent have a teaching certificate or license. Estimates of average years of experience in the field for all child care workers vary by study. One estimate is 4 to 5 years (based on data from

---

[4] This comparison is based on a regression model of wage prediction, consistent with the economics literature, in which education was the dominant factor followed by child care versus other occupations.

[5] This comparison does not include adjustments for the number of working people per household or the average age, education, and work experience of the workers.

the National Institute of Child Health and Human Development [NICHD] Study of Early Child Care and Youth Development); while another is 7 to 12 years (based on data from the National Center for Early Development and Learning Survey and the Head Start Family and Child Experiences Survey). (Brandon emphasized that these figures are for the years of experience gained up to the point at which the survey was given, so the average number of years workers stay in the field would be longer.) Fifty-three to 62 percent of Head Start teachers belong to a professional association (ACF, 2006; FACES, 1997, 2000). Citing data from the 2010 Current Population Survey and 2009 American Community Survey, Brandon reported that approximately 4 to 6 percent of child care workers, and less than 1 percent of family child care workers, belong to a union. Approximately 21 percent of preschool and kindergarten teachers belong to a union.

IMPROVING DATA COLLECTION

The challenge of describing the ECCE workforce makes clear that existing national-level data are inadequate to thoroughly and accurately describe the ECCE workforce, Brandon explained. In particular, no comprehensive and reliable data correspond to the conceptual definition of the workforce he presented. The workshop focused next on what would be required to improve the availability of data, and Brandon described some relevant factors.

A logic model that Brandon (2010) developed for the National Survey of Early Care and Education (NSECE) informed the development of a list of ECCE workforce data elements. The model includes both distal and proximal influences on the quality of early childhood care and education, and their complex interrelationships. For example, distal characteristics, such as demographic characteristics, may affect the professional development a teacher or caregiver attains, which can in turn affect the attitudes and beliefs that shape the quality of caregiving and instruction. Those elements interact with compensation levels. Brandon noted that most of the nationally representative data relate to demographic characteristics of workers and general characteristics of the labor force, factors that may have only distant and indirect relationships to important outcomes. Brandon observed that the factors with the greatest influence on outcomes for children include the more proximal teacher and caregiver characteristics, such as their attitudes, engagement, and skills, as well as the stability of the staff. He added that state and federal policies can affect these characteristics in various ways.

Informed by the logic model, as well as the process of attempting to use existing data to describe the ECCE workforce, Brandon and his colleagues developed a list of potential types and sources of information that would facilitate future efforts by researchers and policy makers. Brandon presented this list of seven broad categories of information:

- Numbers of individuals in the ECCE workforce;
- Distribution of these workers across different child care and educational settings (e.g., center- or home-based, private or public, etc.), ages of children served, and occupational roles (e.g., directors, lead teachers, teaching assistants, aides, specialists);
- Characteristics of the teachers and caregivers (e.g., demographics, qualifications, conditions of employment, compensation and benefits, tenure on the job and in the field);
- Attitudes, attributes, and activities of the teachers and caregivers (e.g., attitudes toward children and parents, job stress and satisfaction, nature of caregiving activities);
- Characteristics of the workplaces (e.g., distribution of staff, supports and professional development offered, turnover, finances, working conditions);
- Distribution of the ECCE workforce and characteristics (e.g., state/county, rural/urban/suburban location, demographic characteristics of children served, prices); and
- Quality of early instruction and caregiving.

A broad range of data sources is needed to be able to answer important policy questions about the ECCE workforce and the ways that it affects child outcomes, Brandon observed. Some information can be found in existing data or planned data collection, such as the NSECE.[6] However, he stressed the need to use multiple sources.

Brandon explained how a federal–state partnership for collecting various types of data might evolve. He described the frequency of data collection, the jurisdictions that might most easily collect each type of data, and the appropriate collection instrument that would be best for each type. "We need to be able to get down to a small geographic level," he observed. "We need to have geographic units that are relevant to policy." One "uber-survey," he explained, could not collect all the kinds of information needed. The Early Childhood Longitudinal Study and the NICHD studies provide useful information, he noted, but more ongoing data collection at the state and community levels is needed as well.[7]

---

[6] The NSECE is a national data collection effort that will update a 1990 study. For more information see http://www.researchconnections.org/childcare/resources/19778.

[7] For more information on these studies, see http://nces.ed.gov/ecls/ and http://www.nichd.nih.gov/, respectively.

With these issues as a context, discussion turned to lessons to be learned from existing data collection efforts.

Learning from National Education Data Systems

The data available about people employed in elementary and secondary education are more complete than what is currently available regarding the ECCE workforce, so K–12 education provides a useful example. As Jerry West, senior fellow at Mathematica Policy Research and former director of the Early Childhood and Household Studies Program at the U.S. Department of Education's NCES, explained, most of the K–12 data are collected by NCES or by states in collaboration with NCES. These studies include federal–state and public–private sector collaborative efforts, which collectively provide a fairly comprehensive picture of education in the United States, as well as information about education in other countries.

The data collection systems cover preschool through postsecondary education and include methods that are designed for different purposes. One broad category is universe surveys, in which data are collected about all of the units within a particular population. The Common Core of Data (CCD), which collects information about all K–12 public schools in the United States, is perhaps the best known of these. The Private School Universe Survey (PSS) is the CCD's counterpart for private schools.[8] These surveys provide basic information about the characteristics of the schools, such as descriptive and demographic information about students and staff, and fiscal data. They also provide the sampling frames (i.e., the enumeration of the populations from which samples should be drawn for analysis of more in-depth questions) for other studies that collect more detailed information about schools, staff, and students.

The sampling studies include cross-sectional surveys (which examine a particular characteristic at a particular time), longitudinal studies (which track changes in a population over time), and hybrids. For example, one component of the Early Childhood Longitudinal Study-Kindergarten Class of 1998–1999 (ECLS-K) focuses on the class of children who were in kindergarten during the 1998–1999 school year.[9] The study collected a variety of information about this population's kindergarten experience and has also followed the children's progress in subsequent years. As a baseline, the ECLS-K sample provides one-time estimates of the characteristics of kindergarten programs and kindergarten teachers nationally.

---

[8] See http://nces.ed.gov/ccd/ for details about the CCD. For details on the PSS, see http://nces.ed.gov/pss/.

[9] See http://nces.ed.gov/ecls/kindergarten.asp for details about the ECLS-K.

TABLE 2-3 National Center for Education Statistics Studies by Reporting Level and Topic

	Reporting Level			
Topic	School	School District	State	National
Student enrollment and characteristics	CCD PSS	CCD	CCD	CCD, PSS, ECLS-K, NHES, CPS, FRSS
Teacher/staff	CCD PSS	CCD	CCD, PSS, SASS	CCD, PSS, SASS, ECLS-K, FRSS
Public school characteristics	CCD	CCD	CCD SASS	CCD, SASS, ECLS-K, FRSS
Private school characteristics	PSS	—	PSS	PSS, SASS, ECLS-K, FRSS
Student outcomes	—	—	NAEP	NAEP, ECLS-K, TIMSS

NOTE: CCD: Common Core of Data; CPS: Current Population Survey; ECLS-K: Early Childhood Longitudinal Study, Kindergarten Class of 1998–1999; FRSS: Fast Response Survey System; NAEP: National Assessment of Educational Progress; NHES: National Household Education Surveys Program; PSS: Private School Universe Survey; SASS: Schools and Staffing Survey; TIMSS: Trends in International Mathematics and Science Study.
SOURCE: West, 2011. Adapted from U.S. Department of Education, National Center for Education Statistics. (2005). *Programs and Plans of the National Center for Education Statistics, 2005 Edition* (NCES 2005113). Washington, DC: National Center for Education Statistics.

Another way to classify the NCES studies is by whether they produce data at the school, district, state, or national level. Table 2-3 arranges key NCES studies by level of reporting and topic. West noted that while all NCES data collection efforts provide some national-level data, only the CCD and its private school counterpart provide school-level data. However, even those studies provide only limited information about teachers, such as the number in each school. The Schools and Staffing Survey (SASS) is a hybrid that uses questionnaires to examine selected topics related to school personnel, and provides more detailed information about teachers.[10]

In thinking about changes or additions to the current system, West noted, one might begin with the type of information that is needed, such as basic information about the size and composition of the ECCE work-

---

[10] See http://nces.ed.gov/surveys/sass/ for details about the SASS.

force, or details about recent trends and changes. Universe surveys can provide such information as the number of teachers or caregivers, the number or percentage of teachers with a B.A., or the number of full- or part-time teachers. "But they don't do a really good job of providing information that allows you to look at the interaction of those characteristics," he added. "If you have a question about what percentage of full-time teachers with a B.A. are teaching or caring for 3-year-olds or the percentage of first-time teachers who are engaged in professional development activities—those types of characteristics are not really well collected through the universe surveys which typically report aggregated data." Answers to these more complex questions often require individual-level data.

The universe surveys are also not very useful for studying emerging issues, so NCES has used the Fast Response Survey System to collect information about issues that cannot be incorporated quickly into ongoing data collection efforts. Fast Response efforts have looked at questions such as how many public schools have a prekindergarten program and the nature of kindergarten teachers' beliefs about children's skills and school readiness. Many questions—such as whether levels of teacher attrition or mobility are changing—require longitudinal data not usually collected in universe surveys.

West noted that the existing system is a collaborative and cooperative one, which is essential because the participant responses are voluntary. Showing how respondents may benefit from the availability of the information is important, he noted. Collaboration is also important because of the need to address discrepancies that may exist between state-level data reporting requirements and those at the federal level. The CCD identifies a data coordinator in each state to coordinate data issues, and a Federal Forum is convened annually that includes representatives from each state to review issues of comparability, changes in data collected, and other data topics. According to West, the PSS requires "buy-in" from "private school organizations to help everyone reach a consensus that there [is] actually value in private school organization as being a part of a federal education data system." NCES nurtures that relationship through an annual meeting with the private school community to address data issues.

Because no one study can answer every important question, West stressed the importance of having a coordinated system. He proposed a system for collecting data on the ECCE workforce, modeled on the NCES approach, as shown in Table 2-4. This table presents a method for selecting an appropriate NCES model on which to base an ECCE data system. This chart shows: (1) type of data collection and purpose for ECCE; (2) NCES model for that type of data; (3) type of data source; (4) sampling unit; and (5) level of data desired (individual versus aggregate). As explained by

TABLE 2-4 A Potential Approach to Data Collection

			Data System		
	Public Program Universe	Private Program Universe	Workforce Survey—Center-Based Programs	Workforce Survey—Home-Based Care	One-Time Surveys—New or Emerging Topics
NCES model	Common Core of Data	Private School Universe Survey	Schools and Staffing Survey	NHES, CPS	Fast Response Survey System
Data source	Administrative records	Survey	Survey	Survey	Survey
Sampling unit	All programs	All programs	Program and teacher samples	Household sample	Varies by topic/issue
Level of data	Aggregate	Aggregate	Individual and aggregate	Individual and aggregate	Varies by topic/issue

NOTE: CPS: Current Population Survey; NCES: National Center for Education Statistics.
SOURCE: West, 2011.

West, "for example ... if you're interested in describing a publicly funded program and you want to have a universe of publicly funded programs ... the model would be the Common Core of Data," which use data from administrative records. West recommended a Schools and Staffing model for center-based ECCE because it provides data both at the program and individual levels. However, he suggested a household survey approach, such as that used in the Current Population Survey, to reach home-based programs. He acknowledged that family child care centers are challenging to categorize in that they could potentially fit either center- or home-based approaches.

This model builds on the work of NCES by including both universe studies that require significant investment and ongoing support as well as sampling studies or fast track or other models for answering different questions. These efforts would require ongoing coordination and collaboration with participants who will take on the burden of responding to regular data collection. He recommended taking the time to learn from existing educational data systems, noting that their history provides many useful lessons and resources.

Learning from a State Example

States vary in how they collect their own data, but Pennsylvania has been at the forefront in the development of a state data system for early childhood care and education. Harriet Dichter, national director of the First Five Years Fund and former secretary of the Pennsylvania Department of Public Welfare, described Pennsylvania's Early Childhood Data System, which the state created to coordinate all of the early childhood programs through the Pennsylvania Office of Child Development and Early Learning (OCDEL). A key element of this task was the development of an integrated data system. This office, the mission of which is to "ensure access to high-quality child and family services," is jointly governed by two state agencies, the Departments of Education and Public Welfare. The four primary responsibilities of OCDEL are:

1. Certification—licensing and inspection of child care facilities;
2. Early intervention services—including technical assistance and early interventions with infants, toddlers, and preschool students;
3. Subsidy services—including parent counseling and referral and Child Care Works (a subsidized child care program); and
4. Early learning services—including public prekindergarten for at-risk preschoolers, full-day kindergarten, Head Start, family support programs, and other programs.

OCDEL staff recognized the need to create an integrated data system that would allow them to monitor their progress and improve quality and outcomes for children. Pennsylvania's Enterprise to Link Information for Children Across Networks (PELICAN) is the information management system developed to meet this goal. It links data from all agencies and programs that serve young children. The Early Learning Network (ELN), one element of PELICAN, is a web-based network for the collection of information about children and the programs that serve them. The data sources are drawn from the many programs serving children and families that are part of PELICAN.

Dichter explained that assessment and accountability were already a part of Pennsylvania's practice: tools used include regular program monitoring and site visits, environmental rating scales and independent third-party review, and performance measures and targets. ELN, a comprehensive data system designed to integrate data about finances, programs, teachers, families, and children, brought standardization across all OCDEL programs. Specifically, the information includes child outcomes, child and family demographics, teacher qualifications and experience, program quality (environmental rating scores), and program demographics, including salaries and benefits for staff. ELN also allows for connections with other data systems, such as those of the Pennsylvania departments of education, child welfare, health, and juvenile justice. Children and teachers are assigned unique secure identification numbers so information can be exchanged without compromising their privacy. The system also integrates professional development data, which helps improve technical assistance to programs and teachers.

ELN has brought a number of other benefits, Dichter explained. It provides feedback to parents about their children's progress, without subjecting the children to multiple assessments. It provides a pool of data that can be used to identify which programs best meet particular kinds of needs, and also provides a basis for evaluating the effectiveness of Pennsylvania's services to young children.

Dichter noted that both PELICAN and ELN were developed in phases over several years, which required creativity, a sustained commitment, and political will from all involved. The developers relied on support from foundations and federal grants, as well as the input of an advisory committee that solicited ideas from all stakeholders. She noted that the existing models and sources of support for the development of these programs were limited. Furthermore, national efforts are sorely needed to develop funding for state-level efforts that can promote consistent definitions and other constructive kinds of standardization.

Looking forward, she observed that the integrated management and data collection system is the foundation for further research on important questions. A comprehensive data system provides a base for addressing critical policy and efficacy questions. For example, data can answer questions regarding:

- Interactions among the learning environment, teacher characteristics, and child development and outcomes;
- The ways in which children's peers and other aspects of the classroom context affect their development;
- The effects of children's and teachers' mobility on the continuity of service and on outcomes for children;
- The effects of receiving multiple services from multiple providers over time;
- The effects of multiple risks for children; and
- Variations in access to high-quality child care by region.

SUMMARY

Brandon summarized key messages from these presentations and discussions, observing that a large, complex, and well-coordinated federal structure provides comparable data across all occupations and industries in the United States. The ECCE field needs to decide the extent to which the benefits of participating in this structure outweigh the difficulties associated with fitting complex and overlapping occupational roles within it. The possibility of comparing data across multiple contexts is an important consideration, he stressed. At the same time, the coordination of federal education and state data at the K–12 level provides a useful model for the ECCE field to examine. Data collection efforts in education have demonstrated the importance of cooperation among federal and state agencies as well as public and private enterprises. The Pennsylvania example illustrated the extremely valuable role that integrated data collection can play in supporting sound policy and improvements in quality in ECCE. All three multicomponent systems demonstrate several key points, he noted:

- No one specific data collection effort can meet all needs;
- All require collaboration; and
- All must develop over time.

However, he added, much work is needed both to capitalize on existing systems and to develop new ones at the state and federal levels that can provide the comprehensive data the ECCE field needs. At present, a participant noted, the registries and workforce data systems developed by states as part of their professional development and quality improvement efforts are the main sources of workforce data for program developers and policy makers. As participants also noted, although capitalizing on existing systems is important, so is capturing the reality of ECCE as it is practiced. Most existing data systems focus on describing and measuring the activities of individuals, while the field often emphasizes serving the needs of children through team-based and collaborative efforts. The best way to reconcile these two goals will require further discussion of the merits of different data models and measurement approaches.

3

Economic Perspectives on the Early Childhood Care and Education Workforce

Market forces shape the availability, quality, and price of early childhood care and education (ECCE). Economic analyses illuminate the way this market operates and provides a context for evaluating policies and interventions designed to improve and support the workforce and improve the quality of care. Caregivers, teachers, parents, and providers all respond to numerous interrelated market forces, as well as other influences. Consequently, as policy makers decide whether and how to intervene to achieve important goals—such as improving school readiness, closing achievement gaps, reducing school failure, reducing crime, and increasing graduation rates—economic analyses can point to both intended and unintended consequences, and provide empirical evidence to demonstrate the potential value gained from particular types of investments in early childhood care and education. David Blau, professor of economics at Ohio State University, provided an overview of the way economists think about this market and identified some lessons for policy makers. Lynn Karoly, senior economist at the RAND Corporation, described economists' efforts to measure the short- and long-term costs and benefits of investing in ECCE.

THE EARLY CHILDHOOD LABOR MARKET

The ECCE workforce has special importance in American society, Blau noted, because policy makers, parents, and researchers care about the development and well-being of young children. Compensation for the

ECCE workforce, as well as benefits, working conditions, training, education, and opportunities for advancement, are important for this group—as they are for workers in any occupation or industry. Blau observed that although these workers have special importance because of the influence they have on children, in the United States our society relies largely on market forces to determine the quantity in which care is available, its quality, and its price. As the ECCE field considers how to craft policies that improve access, availability, and quality of care, researchers need to understand the market factors that affect how parents select or change their care arrangements.

Demand in the early childhood market is a function of how parents select their child care arrangements. Many factors affect these decisions. Parents' beliefs, preferences, income levels, and constraints (e.g., working hours or transportation) all influence their willingness and ability to purchase child care at alternative prices. Parents will consider the type of care arrangement (e.g., center, family child care, nanny); the developmental quality of the care arrangement; and its convenience and reliability. From an economic perspective, the key point is their willingness to substitute different types and quality of care arrangements in response to different prices. Thus, supply of education and care encompasses the full range of types of care available, even if these types are regulated, funded, or viewed separately by those in the field. Evidence suggests, Blau explained, that parents have a "moderate willingness to substitute" (Blau and Hagy, 1998). In other words, parents are not ready to abandon a care arrangement in response to a small increase in price, but as the price of developmentally appropriate and stimulating care increases relative to alternatives, they are willing to make trade-offs.

The supply of child care, in turn, is influenced by what economists call the "technology" of producing the care and the prices of the inputs—primarily the cost of employing staff with particular levels of skill and qualifications. These factors affect providers' willingness to offer child care at alternative prices according to quality, type, and location. A key aspect of supply is the degree of flexibility of the technology: Is there more than one way to produce a given level of quality of child care? Blau indicated that considerable flexibility exists in this field: "Must you have, for example, a director with a master's degree in early childhood education, a lead teacher with a bachelor's degree, an assistant with a certain level of education and training, a group size of a defined level, and a child/staff ratio" in order to provide child care of high developmental quality? Observational studies that compare child care centers that all meet certain defined levels of quality have shown that they meet these levels in a variety of ways, Blau explained (Blau, 1997, 2000). International comparisons reinforce this point. In France, for example, the child care system is very well-regarded, though group sizes and staff-to-child ratios would violate regulations in most U.S. states (Richardson and Marx, 1989). For example, group sizes of 3- to 6-year old children in France's universal preschool program averaged 25.5 students per class with 1 teacher and 1 assistant, as of 2001–2002 (OECD, 2006). French policy pays close attention to teacher training, however, which may be a less expensive way to meet quality goals.

Another key determinant of supply is what economists call the degree of input specialization—in this case the degree to which the skills of ECCE workers are useful and in demand in other occupations. Here the evidence suggests that the skills needed in early child care and education are not highly specialized, and are valued in other occupations. As a consequence, the labor supply in the child care sector has relatively high elasticity because the wages available are low compared with wages in other sectors that require similar skills. For example, early childhood teachers who possess the required qualifications may choose to leave a preschool position for higher wages in a K–12 teaching position.

Together, the supply of and demand for child care interact to determine the market equilibrium—the prices at which child care of alternative types and quality can be purchased. Thus, consumers' willingness to substitute one care arrangement for another and the flexibility of the technology jointly determine the outcomes observed in the market. However, other forces may impinge on the child care market. Government policy, in particular, may influence the demand for different types of child care or levels of quality by imposing standards and regulations or by providing subsidized care.

Labor is the main input in the production of child care, Blau observed, and the demand by providers for child care workers with different skill levels derives from the demand by parents for child care of different types and quality. Empirical analyses of the labor market for child care show that:

- High-quality (developmentally stimulating) care is costly, and consumers are moderately sensitive to price. Many consumers feel "priced out" of the market for high-quality care, which limits the demand for skilled staff (Blau and Mocan, 2002);
- The supply of child care workers is relatively elastic, so an increase in demand for child care does not exert much upward pressure on wages for child care workers (Blau, 1993, 2001); and
- Skilled staff have good opportunities in other occupations and sectors, so turnover is high (Blau, 1992, 2001).

Blau considered whether these findings show evidence of market failure and thus provide a rationale for the government to intervene in the market to improve outcomes. He defined market failure as a situation in which the quantity of a service (or product) that is available based on the equilibrium between supply and demand is not equal to the quantity society would deem optimal—in this case the market would have failed if the supply of high-quality child care was not sufficient to meet the needs of children and families. Unfortunately, economists cannot identify the socially optimal amount of high-quality child care. First, strong evidence of the long-term benefits of child care is relatively scarce—even though many studies exist (see Costs and Benefits of Investing in Early Childhood Education in this chapter). In Blau's view they do not yield sufficient empirical support for firm or precise conclusions. Second, the socially optimal level is determined in part by value judgments.

Data on outcomes could provide further insight into the issue of market failure, Blau observed. Figure 3-1 shows trends in families' expenditures on child care, drawn from a household survey (the Survey of Income and Program Participation [SIPP]). These data indicate that the real (inflation-adjusted) average weekly expenditure on child care per family that pays for care has increased by about 3.3 percent per year over 20 years. The total number of families paying for care has also increased, by about 2.9 percent per year on average. Together, those two changes imply an average annual growth rate of 6.3 percent per year in total child care expenditures over a 20-year period.

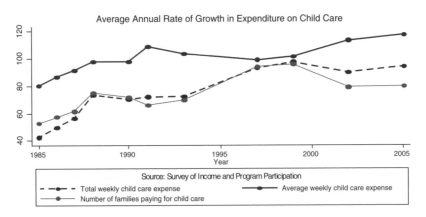

FIGURE 3-1 Trends in family child care expenditure.
NOTE: Total weekly child care expense in units of $10M; average weekly child care expense in real inflation-adjusted dollars; number of families paying for child care in units of 100,000; all dollar amounts in 2009 dollars.
SOURCE: Blau, 2011.

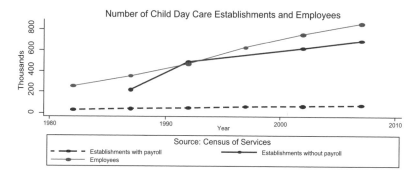

FIGURE 3-2 Trends in the number of establishments and employees.
SOURCE: Blau, 2011.

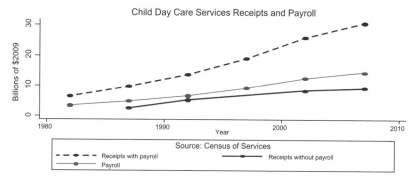

FIGURE 3-3 Trends in receipts and payroll.
SOURCE: Blau, 2011.

At the same time, data from the U.S. Census Bureau's Census of Service Industries for a recent 25-year period show that the number of child care establishments with payrolls has increased at an average annual rate of 3.6 percent; the number of employees has increased 4.8 percent per year; and the number of establishments without payrolls (individuals caring for children at home) has grown by 9 percent per year (see Figure 3-2). Figure 3-3 shows rapid growth in the receipts taken in by these establishments and in their payroll expenditures.

The Occupational Employment Statistics (OES) published by the Bureau of Labor Statistics (BLS) show that the number of child care workers grew at an average rate of 4.6 percent annually during a recent 10-year period, compared to a lower (1.4 percent) annual growth rate among the number of preschool teachers. Total employment in all occupations grew by just 0.3 percent per year on average during that same period. In contrast to rapid growth in the size of the child care sector, hourly wages for child care workers have grown by just 0.5 percent per year on average (0.8 percent for preschool teachers, as compared with wages for all workers, which have grown by 0.7 percent).[1]

These data paint a consistent and surprising picture, Blau explained. Why did the sharp increase in demand for child care not result in larger increases in wages for the ECCE workforce? Blau suggested that the primary reason is the highly elastic supply of labor for child care work. For example, he noted, many female immigrants from developing countries have few good employment options in the United States and are willing to work in child care for relatively low wages. Thus an increase in the supply of these workers is likely to depress wages. One might expect that this would apply mainly to the relatively low-quality segment of the child care market, but because parents are moderately sensitive to price, it is likely that more highly skilled child care workers' wages would also be depressed, as researchers Hock and Furtado (2009) found. They report that low-skilled immigrants grew from 6.1 percent of the working population in the United States in 1980 to 10.1 percent in 2000. This trend contributed to the decline in child care wage rate, compared with what might have occurred in the absence of an increase in immigration. The decline affected child care workers throughout the skill distribution.

While frustrating to many, these trends alone do not imply market failure, Blau explained. But he sees other significant problems in the child care market. In his view, the failure is not on the supply side of the equation, but on the demand side. Parents do not have sufficient willingness (or capacity) to pay for high-quality child care. High-quality care benefits not only individual children, but also society in general (this point is discussed further below), yet parents tend not to consider the social benefit. In response to participant comments, Blau acknowledged practical limits to what some parents can pay. Although parents could take out loans to pay for child care and education, for example, as they do for college, few are likely to take that step, at least without substantial evidence that doing so would be critical to their own children's development.

Evidence of the benefits of high-quality preschool for disadvantaged children provides strong reasons to suggest that society should pay the cost of improving their access to high-quality care and education. The case for supporting children and families who are not disadvantaged is more difficult, Blau explained. The empirical evidence for the long-term

---

[1] A participant suggested that the constraints of child care subsidies or the inclusion of paid relatives in the analysis could potentially distort the nature of the overall picture.

benefits of high-quality child care, as compared with mediocre child care, for typical middle-class children is more limited.

Making the case for specific types of public intervention is difficult without strong empirical evidence, Blau noted. An issue from the K–12 education context illustrates the point. Abundant evidence exists that effective teachers have a significant impact on student learning, Blau explained. However, little evidence exists that specific qualifications, such as degrees earned, training, and certification can identify the successful teachers. Thus, proponents of the social benefit of increasing spending to improve teacher effectiveness in schools encounter persistent skepticism (Hanushek, 2011; Hanushek and Rivkin, 2007).

Blau's conclusion is that market intervention will be most successful if it targets the source of the failure, which he views as the relatively low demand for high-quality care. Interventions such as subsidies for high-quality care and public awareness campaigns could increase demand, which could, in turn, raise wages for skilled staff. Addressing the supply side by, for example, imposing more stringent education and training requirements, or providing subsidies to encourage training and boost wages, is less likely to be successful, he argued. Regulations that do not come with financial support for improving quality often have unintended negative consequences. For example, if a center is faced with the requirement to have smaller groups and more staff, it may only be able to achieve that result by reducing wages. Wage or training subsidies do not work well when the labor supply is very elastic, he explained, because workers still have higher paying alternatives.

The realities of the marketplace, Blau concluded, show that the choices that parents, caregivers and teachers, and employers make, as well as the choices policy makers make by allocating public funding or imposing regulations, all affect the child care market in both positive and negative ways. While the market may not have failed, in a technical sense, he suggested, the problems with available child care options could be more easily resolved if all actors in the system had a better understanding of the nature and benefits of high-quality care.

COSTS AND BENEFITS OF INVESTING IN
EARLY CHILDHOOD EDUCATION

Interest in the empirical evidence of the short- and long-term returns to investments made in early childhood care and education is increasing, Karoly explained. Resources are scarce, both for foundations and other private entities that could contribute in this area, as well as for public agencies. Funders in all categories are increasingly emphasizing results-based accountability. Thus, these groups benefit from data that not only demonstrate immediate program benefits, but also show how long-term benefits translate into specific savings to governments, including data that estimate the dollar value of benefits to society. Data that indicate that a $1 investment will yield a return of $X can be very powerful in providing a basis for choosing one program over another or making decisions about current or future program spending in general, she noted.[2]

Karoly described several different analytic approaches to this challenge:

- Cost analysis, which measures only costs, not outcomes;
- Cost-effectiveness analysis, in which the impact for one outcome is measured, in natural units, relative to costs;
- Cost–savings analysis, in which the benefits (and costs) to the government of all outcomes are valued in dollars and compared with costs; and
- Benefit–cost analysis, in which the benefits (and costs) for society—for both program participants and nonparticipants—of all outcomes are valued in dollars and compared with costs.

Each approach begins with careful calculation of program costs, relative to the status quo or to some other option. The next step, cost-effectiveness analysis, asks what it costs to achieve a particular degree of change in one particular outcome. This could be done separately for more than one outcome, but it does not involve assigning a dollar value to the outcomes. Cost–savings analysis and benefit–cost analysis both entail assigning a dollar value to the full range of program outcomes, which is a more difficult challenge (see NRC and IOM, 2009).

These tools have been used only to a limited degree in the early childhood context, Karoly explained. Recently, however, researchers have begun to use them to examine the economic returns on investments in specific programs for children from birth to age 5. A 2005 RAND Corporation study (Karoly et al., 2005) examined 20 interventions for this age group and found that 19 of them showed favorable outcomes for participating children or their parents. These programs are listed in Table 3-1, where they are arranged to distinguish between programs that focused on home visiting and parental education and those that provided early childhood education.

Karoly presented the results of benefit–cost analyses for six of these programs (Karoly, 2011a). The ratios of benefits to costs shown in Figure 3-4, some based on short-term follow-up data and some on long-term

---

[2] Karoly noted several sources of further detail on these issues: Karoly (2011a); Karoly et al. (2005); Kilburn and Karoly (2008).

TABLE 3-1 Early Childhood Interventions with Demonstrated Favorable Outcomes

Six Effective Programs Have Associated Benefit–Cost Analysis (BCA)	
Home Visiting/Parent Education	Early Childhood Education/ Combination
Dare to Be You	Abecedarian Program*
Developmental Supporting Care: Newborn Individualized Developmental Care and Assessment Program (DSC/NIDCAP)	Chicago Child-Parent Centers (CPC)*
Home Instruction for Parents of Preschool Youngsters (HIPPY USA)*	Comprehensive Child Development Program (CCDP)
Incredible Years	Early Head Start
Nurse Family Partnership (NFP)*	Early Training Program
Parents as Teacher	Head Start
Project CARE (Carolina Approach to Responsive Education)	Houston Parent-Child Development Center (PCDC)
Reach Out and Read	Infant Health and Development Program (IHDP)* Oklahoma Universal Preschool
	Perry Preschool Project*
	Syracuse Family Development Research Program

* Programs for which benefit–cost analysis has been conducted.
SOURCE: Karoly, 2011b. Based on Karoly et al., 2005.

results, range from no positive economic returns (Infant Health and Development Program [IHDP]) to 16.1:1 (Perry Preschool Project at the age 40 follow-up). Karoly drew several conclusions from these data. First, regarding the IHDP, the one program in the analysis that did not show positive economic returns, she cautioned that such results can occur for several reasons. "Many of the benefits that come out of these programs, particularly when you're looking at the early stages of the follow-up ... are harder to quantify in economic terms," she observed. Longer term benefits to which the analyst did not assign a dollar value may emerge later. She also noted that it was not just the small-scale demonstration

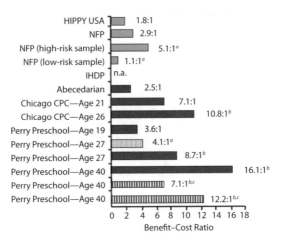

FIGURE 3-4 Results of benefit–cost analyses for six programs.
NOTE: A benefit–cost ratio is the ratio of the present discounted value of total benefits to society as a whole (participants and the rest of society) divided by present discounted value of program costs. The discount rate is 3 percent unless otherwise noted. The value of reducing intangible crime victim costs are excluded unless otherwise noted. CPC: child-parent centers; HIPPY USA: Home Instruction for Parents of Preschool Youngsters; IHDP: Infant Health and Development Program; NFP: Nurse-Family Partnership.
[a] Discount rate is 4 percent.
[b] Includes value of reduced intangible crime victim costs.
[c] Reported range of estimates under alternative assumptions regarding the economic cost of crime.
SOURCE: Karoly, 2011b. Based on Karoly, 2011a.

programs that generated positive economic returns. Critics sometimes dismiss the economic benefits shown by the Perry Preschool Project, for example, on the grounds that it would be difficult to replicate. The results for HIPPY USA: Home Instruction for Parents of Preschool Youngsters (1.8:1) and the Chicago Child-Parent Centers program (7.1:1 at age 21 and 10.8:1 at age 26) counter that point, however. Moreover, it is not just the most expensive, intensive programs that show favorable benefit–cost ratios, as HIPPY USA also demonstrates. On the other hand, it may be that programs that target children with the greatest needs show larger returns compared with those that serve more advantaged children. Perhaps most important, she noted, is that effective programs with longer term follow-up tend to show larger returns than those that only had shorter term follow-up results. That is, the more data that are accumulated, and the greater the time for benefits to emerge, the greater the quantifiable value of the return on investment.

Karoly cautioned that these results cannot be used to compare the programs directly because they include a mix of types of interventions, as well as of lengths of follow-up, outcomes measured, target populations, and analytic methods. These results are important, she noted, because they demonstrate that investments in early childhood programs that are of high quality and are implemented well provide concrete benefits. Indeed, she observed that the researchers were conservative in their long-term estimates of benefits, and that it is probable that the economic value of a number of these programs is greater than the analyses indicate at this point.

Karoly enumerated significant challenges to this type of analysis, however. First, it requires rigorous analysis of the incremental costs, in comparison to a baseline, and programs do not always keep careful records of all of the costs of implementing a new program. The costs of the alternative approaches that would have been used in the absence of the new program may also be difficult to capture. Second, rigorous evaluations—either experimental or rigorous quasi-experimental studies—are needed to establish program effects.[3]

The benefits of these types of programs may include effects for both parents and children and for society at large in a broad range of domains (e.g., education, employment, mental and emotional health, involvement with the justice system), some of which are easier to measure than others. Placing a dollar value on benefits in these areas poses challenges as well. The field is just beginning to develop standardized methods that will make comparisons more valid, she added.

Despite these challenges, Karoly advocates greater use of benefit–cost analysis and cost-effectiveness analysis in the early childhood sphere, and she highlighted areas where this approach could be especially valuable. Cost-effectiveness or benefit–cost analysis of marginal changes in program features, policy alternatives, and specific interventions could all be very useful. For example, if a state legislature wishes to improve early learning and considers increasing spending by $500 per child, one could use cost-effectiveness analysis to determine whether a particular outcome for children could be produced for that price. Alternatively, one could assess a variety of interventions—such as changing group sizes or ratios, or increasing education requirements for teachers—to determine which approach would provide the most valuable benefit. Another pos-

---

[3] Quasi-experimental designs are those used where randomized controlled designs are not possible, practical, or ethical. They use alternate statistical procedures to isolate causal effects.

sibility would be to compare several possible approaches to improving professional development for teachers to see which would produce the largest gains, either in terms of child development or quantified dollar benefits. Producing this type of information for supporting policy decisions, Karoly believes, will require that cost-effectiveness and benefit–cost analysis be incorporated into the next generation of research on early childhood program design and interventions.

SUMMARY

In summary, Blau indicated that despite the tremendous increase in the demand for child care, wages for workers have remained relatively flat, due in part to the elastic supply of people willing to work in ECCE for relatively low wages, as well as their high rates of turnover. These factors coupled with relatively low demand for high-quality care make increasing wages difficult. This dilemma has led some to consider whether and how government might play a role in addressing the cycle of low compensation and high turnover. As Karoly's presentation showed, one reason that governments might elect to play a role in addressing these problems is because of the demonstrated positive economic returns of high-quality care and education, particularly for disadvantaged children. Effective care and education depends in large part on having a workforce with the right combination of skills, attitudes, behaviors, and characteristics that functions within supportive workplaces (topics examined in further detail in Chapter 4). According to Karoly, new approaches to calculating the costs and benefits of child care are promising and may prove particularly useful for policy makers in weighing the most effective investments in the early childhood care and education workforce.

4

How the Workforce Affects Children

Caregivers and teachers form important relationships with the children in their care. Through these relationships, critical behaviors, such as language use with children, emotional tone and warmth, responsiveness and sensitivity, and intentional teaching, all directly affect child development and have longer term effects on later schooling and social-emotional adjustment (NRC, 2001; NRC and IOM, 2000). Evidence is mounting that the behaviors of teachers and caregivers are important; however, determining how to identify, prepare, and support those who practice these desirable skills is more challenging. Researchers and policy makers both have an interest in determining which characteristics (e.g., amount of training, years of experience, possession of a college degree) are associated with the practices that promote healthy child development, as well as how to produce these practices on a large scale across the early childhood care and education (ECCE) workforce, a topic addressed in Chapter 5. This chapter includes presentations and discussion of the research on these important behaviors and characteristics of the workforce, the effects of working conditions of the workforce, as well as the implications of these working conditions for teachers, caregivers, and children.

EFFECTS OF THE WORKFORCE ON CHILD DEVELOPMENT

A great deal of research has focused on the relations between children's experiences in non-parental care and their short- and long-term development. Though a complete review of these data was beyond the scope of this workshop, the National Institute of Child Health and Human Development (NICHD) Study of Early Child Care and Youth Development[1] is a landmark study of these early experiences. The study included a full range of settings and income groups and serves as a rich source of data regarding the effects of the workforce on child development. Aletha Huston, the Priscilla Pond Flawn Regents Professor of Child Development at the University of Texas at Austin, described some of the findings from this work.

This longitudinal study involves a number of research teams and has followed children in 10 locations since 1991, collecting data on those who were in any type of non-maternal child care for more than 10 hours a week. The researchers observed the child care when the children were ages 6, 15, 24, 36, and 54 months. The observers recorded minute-by-minute documentation of the child's experiences and used rating scales to assess aspects of the caregiving environment. Researchers also collected data on the caregivers,[2] covering issues such as their training and education, beliefs and attitudes, reasons for becoming child care workers, and psychological well-being.

Huston used a model of the relations among caregivers' characteristics, the features of the caregiving environment, the behavior of the adults and children in the caregiving setting, and outcomes for children to organize her discussion (see Figure 4-1). Researchers have examined these constructs and the relations among them to study interactions and differences that may occur among children of varying ages.

For infants, the researchers used a measure of "positive caregiving quality," a composite of caregiver sensitivity, positive regard for the child, cognitive stimulation, engagement, and other features, to assess the quality of the adult–child interactions in the child care setting. They observed higher quality when several factors were in place:

- Low child-to-adult ratio;
- Small group size;
- Caregivers with non-traditional child-rearing beliefs;[3] and
- High-quality physical environment (e.g., amount and types of various materials, health and safety features).

---

[1] See http://www.nichd.nih.gov/research/supported/seccyd/overview.cfm for details about the NICHD.

[2] This section of the report uses the term "caregivers" as it was used in the workshop presentation.

[3] This characteristic is also sometimes called a child-centered approach, Huston explained, and it refers to the caregiver's conviction that giving the child opportunities to develop autonomy, express feelings, and make decisions while still setting limits is important.

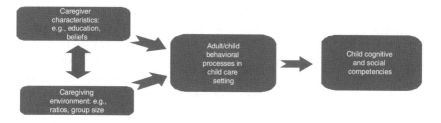

FIGURE 4-1 Model of early childhood education.
SOURCE: Malerba, 2005.

These factors, Huston explained, had stronger relations to outcomes than did caregivers' experience, training, and formal education.

For toddlers (ages 15 to 36 months), the importance of the child-to-caregiver ratio for predicting quality declined, and by age 3 the ratio was not related to quality. The degree to which non-traditional beliefs contributed to quality increased in importance with the age of the children, and the importance of caregiver education also increased, though training did not add much predictive value.

Huston also reported on an analysis of caregivers who worked with 2-year-olds, in which the researchers identified five caregiver characteristics as important to outcomes for children (Malerba, 2005):

- Education, formal training, and non-traditional beliefs about child rearing;
- Years of experience and age;
- Conscientiousness about the job and commitment to caring for young children, and low levels of depression;
- Finding personal rewards in the job; and
- Professionalism and recent training (among family child care providers only).

Of these, caregiver non-traditional beliefs, professionalism, and concerns about caring for children all predicted observed positive engagement with children on the caregivers' part, but features of the environment (e.g., ratios, healthy practices) were stronger predictors. In child care homes, the caregiver characteristics were weak predictors. Features of the environment (e.g., ratio, having a schedule) were also strong predictors here.

These researchers examined the relationships between meeting external quality standards and positive outcomes for children (NICHD, 1999). They determined the extent to which centers met external standards for quality care established by professional or regulatory organizations, which address features such as ratio, group size, caregiver education level, and caregiver training. The quality criteria do appear to be important. For example, low child-to-adult ratios for children at ages 2 and 3 predict both high levels of positive social behavior and low levels of problem behavior in the children. For 3-year-olds, caregiver education and training predicted school readiness, high language comprehension, and low levels of behavior problems. Analyses that examined the experiences of children at 54 months also found that caregivers' education, training, and ratios were associated with children's development of cognitive and social competencies. For children in family child care, the caregiver's non-authoritarian beliefs and education were both associated with children's cognitive skills.

Huston summarized the key findings from these analyses:

- For the youngest children, the structural features of the environment, particularly the child-to-adult ratios, often outweigh caregiver characteristics.
- The relative importance of caregiver characteristics and ratios changes from infancy to preschool settings; ratio is especially important in the first 2 or 3 years. Caregiver beliefs and training are especially important for older children.
- Non-traditional, child-centered beliefs about child rearing mediate at least part of the benefits of caregiver education and formal training, although the causal links are not understood. Possibilities are that people who have those beliefs are more likely to seek education, or that education and training can influence those beliefs, for example, or that both are true.

Huston suggested that policy makers should consider children's ages in defining quality of care, and should develop standards that are appropriate for different age groups. Training might be more effective if it dealt directly with beliefs and attitudes about child rearing, rather than just curriculum and strategies. At the same time, even the best trained caregivers are limited by the structural and environmental constraints of their settings. Policy makers may wish that improved training could compensate for high ratios for the youngest children, but the evidence seems to suggest otherwise. Thus, she observed, "if we are really thinking about attempts to upgrade the workforce, then it involves upgrading the environments in which people work, as well as upgrading their skills."

One participant noted that the results discussed were not derived from experimental or quasi-experimental designs and that, despite extensive controls for family and child characteristics, they do not support causal inferences. For example, some of the positive association between a particular teacher or center characteristic and a child outcome could be the result of unmeasured factors that lead parents to place their child in high-quality care, and that would have led to good outcomes for the child even in the absence of high-quality care.

The Impact of Teacher Qualifications

In recent years, a great deal of attention in research and policy has focused on teacher qualifications as a means of identifying those best prepared to deliver high-quality experiences for children. Specifically, research has sought to determine the relationship of teacher degrees and/ or amount or types of training to the quality of their caregiving and teaching, as well as to children's outcomes. Debate in the field about whether early childhood teachers should be required to hold bachelor's (B.A.) degrees has been fueled in part by mixed research findings on the topic (Early et al., 2007; Helburn, 1995; Whitebook and Ryan, 2011). Two researchers, Margaret Burchinal, senior scientist at the Frank Porter Graham Child Development Institute at the University of North Carolina, and Steve Barnett, codirector of the National Institute for Early Education Research, who have examined this topic in detail, presented research findings and their views.

High-quality child care experiences are consistently related to better outcomes for children in general, and especially for low-income children, Burchinal observed. Experimental studies have shown that the effects of at least moderate- to high-quality care are evident through adulthood. High-quality care, she explained, involves close teacher–child relationships, frequent sensitive interactions between the child and the teacher, high-quality instruction, and respectful and effective behavior management. High-quality care also involves other features, such as rich physical environment.

Early research suggested that a B.A. degree successfully identified teachers who provided high-quality care (Burchinal et al., 2000; Helburn, 1995; Whitebook et al., 1990). Policy makers responded with requirements that teachers have a B.A., and teaching certificates for early childhood were established accordingly. Head Start instituted a policy requiring that 50 percent of teachers in a center have a B.A., and many state prekindergarten programs had similar policies.

However, Burchinal explained, more recent work (Early et al., 2007; Whitebook and Ryan, 2011) has challenged the findings about the relevance of a B.A. She suggested several possible explanations. Cohort effects could explain the differences between the groups who had B.A. degrees and worked in early childhood at the time of the early studies and those who have that profile now. Differences in the measures and methods the researchers used is another possible explanation, so Burchinal and her colleagues conducted a secondary analysis of data from seven large preschool projects, including evaluations of prekindergarten programs, longitudinal studies of community programs, and others (Early et al., 2007). They used consistent definitions of teacher education levels (e.g., type of degree and certification), and standard measures of quality and child outcomes (e.g., Early Childhood Environmental Rating Scale [ECERS], Woodcock-Johnson Applied Problems).[4] They also used consistent analytic methods to account for missing data and nesting of children in classrooms. Across 27 separate analyses, they found 5 that showed statistically significant effects favoring possession of a B.A., 4 that showed a benefit for possession of any degree, and 2 that showed a benefit for teacher certification.

In Burchinal's view, the findings show that measures of child care quality or child outcomes were not consistently related to any of the ways of measuring teacher education. The researchers considered possible explanations for these findings. One possibility is that many of the preservice programs for teachers included in the studies were new and their instruction might not have reflected current research regarding effective practices. This hypothesis is supported by a 2008 web-based survey of programs that provide degrees in ECCE. The researchers found that although these programs relied on standards for both coursework and fieldwork, few were actually focusing on developing supportive teacher–child relationships, and few included research in their teaching about practices (Hyson et al., 2008). For example, only 46 percent of the teacher preparation programs cited teachers' interactions with children as an important focus. In general, the programs were understaffed and heavily reliant on part-time faculty. Thus, the quality of these teacher preparation programs appears to be very uneven. They are typically small and underfunded, and have seen large enrollment increases without commensurate increases in resources to meet the demand.

The good news, Burchinal noted, is that some training programs for existing teachers can be effective at improving quality and child outcomes. A meta-analysis of studies of training programs that focused on direct teaching practices or interactions with children found that programs that were tightly tailored and used manuals to address a specific issue had positive effects (Fukkink and Lont, 2007). Other work, Burchinal added, supports the idea that intensive training programs with clearly defined curriculums and coaching—for example, using defined curriculums, video observations, and onsite mentoring for both entry-level and

---

[4] ECERS is a rating scale for early childhood programs; the Woodcock-Johnson is a tool for measuring cognitive and academic skills.

more experienced staff—can be effective (Clements and Sarama, 2007; Dickinson and Caswell, 2007; Lonigan and Whitehurst, 1998; Pianta et al., 2008; Powell et al., 2010; Wasik et al., 2010).

In summary, Burchinal believes the research does not currently support the B.A. as a critical factor in the quality of early childhood teachers. "Quality can be improved," she suggested, "when teachers receive carefully selected and implemented professional development, either during pre- or in-service training. We should move beyond a focus on whether the lead teacher has a B.A. to a focus on the content and quality of the higher education program." Additional research on the specific course requirements or internship practices, approaches to induction of new teachers, coaching, and other strategies, she added, could help pinpoint the best ways to improve the quality of teachers and outcomes for children. She believes that combining effective higher education with onsite induction and coordinated professional development are the most promising avenues for progress.

Barnett provided another perspective on the evidence regarding teacher quality and qualifications. He referenced an article he coauthored with several colleagues, including Burchinal, which addressed key policy questions about the effects of preschool education (Pianta et al., 2009). In that article, the authors assert that the ways that teachers interact with children and their ability to effectively implement appropriate curriculums may matter more to child outcomes than their qualifications, in part because these behaviors "do not appear to be produced in a reliable manner by typical teacher preparation" (Pianta et al., 2009, p. 50). Informed by this work, Barnett offered his own views on an alternative set of questions that should guide future data collection and analysis:

- How do children's learning and development vary with teacher characteristics?
- What teacher characteristics are needed to achieve goals for early childhood care and education (e.g., to close 50 or 75 percent of the learning gap for children entering kindergarten)?
- Do the effects of teacher characteristics vary with other program features and policies, and with the populations served?
- Under what conditions do teacher qualifications make (or not make) a substantive difference?

On the question of the characteristics teachers need to meet desired goals, Barnett noted that the National Research Council (2001) report, *Eager to Learn: Educating Our Preschoolers*, provided a good definition of what prekindergarten teachers need to know (see Box 4-1) and offered a valuable basis for this kind of research. Different types of research studies

---

BOX 4-1
Skills and Knowledge Prekindergarten Teachers Need

- Current understanding of how to put up-to-date knowledge of teaching, learn-ing, and child development into practice—particularly specific foundational knowledge of socio-emotional development and mathematics, science, linguis-tics, and literature;
- Capacity to provide rich conceptual experiences that promote growth in spe-cific content areas (e.g., mathematics, science) and in broad domains (e.g., language, cognition);
- Effective teaching strategies, including, but not limited to, new knowledge re-garding how children learn to read;
- Capacity to identify appropriate content for preschool children;
- Assessment procedures to inform instruction;
- Teaching practices for children who are not fluent in English, come from dif-ferent cultural/social backgrounds, have disabilities, or differ from the normal range of development; and
- Capacity to work with parents and other family members.

SOURCE: Adapted from NRC, 2001.

---

can be useful, he observed. Research on effective parenting, studies of program effectiveness, natural variation studies that examine children before and after their early learning experiences, and studies of changes over time resulting from policy shifts (e.g., changes in requirements for teachers) all may contribute useful knowledge.

One recent study provides an overview of research on program char-acteristics' effects on children, though Barnett noted that the measures of teacher qualifications are fairly crude because the sampled studies did not all use the same coding procedures (Camilli et al., 2010). This study found positive effects for programs that incorporated intentional teaching (i.e., purposeful and planned activities to achieve specific educational objectives) and also for programs in which children received significant amounts of one-on-one attention. Like Burchinal, Barnett noted that some meta-analyses show small effects for possession of a B.A. (Early et al., 2007; Kelley and Camilli, 2007).

Looking at the available findings another way, Barnett noted that the prekindergarten programs that have produced significant gains for children, particularly in randomized trials, all shared several factors: well-educated teachers (B.A. or higher); adequate compensation (comparable to public school salaries); strong curriculum and professional develop-ment; small classes and reasonable teacher-to-child ratios; strong supervision, monitoring, and review; and both high standards and continuous improvement. Without all of these features, Barnett observed, a program would be unlikely to achieve the same results: "We don't see one that produced great results—like Abecedarian, Perry Preschool, or Chicago Child-Parent Centers—that did not have all of those characteristics."

This general finding is important, but Barnett believes existing research has significant limitations. First, no randomized controlled studies of teacher characteristics have been completed. Second, the measures of child learning and development that are used as dependent variables are "narrow and highly imperfect." He noted that tools such as the Woodcock-Johnson test (see earlier footnote, this section) are limited measures of children's educational outcomes and are not likely to be good measures of teachers' contributions to those outcomes. Similarly, rating scales such as the ECERS are useful measures of classroom and program environments, but they are not sophisticated enough to capture the differences between poor- and good-quality teaching. On the other hand, the independent variables are heterogeneous. Teacher degrees may reflect quite rigorous preparation or may be available from a "diploma mill." The same is true for teacher in-service training and professional development, he added; they vary so much that the benefits of excellent programs might be obscured in data that also include poor-quality programs.

At the same time, teachers and students are not independent—children are not randomly assigned to preschool classrooms and teachers are not randomly assigned to programs, and these selection biases significantly complicate studies of the contributions teachers make to children's outcomes. Teachers who work together also influence one another. A study that focused on the lead teachers without taking into account the influence of coteachers would likely miss the effects of their interactions. Moreover, the varying ways in which centers' or states' policies regarding staffing are implemented may also bias results.

Another set of issues relates to the factors that influence how much teacher education is typical in a program. The curriculum, the director's views, the availability of services and supports (e.g., child study teams or coaching), and the program's educational goals are likely to affect the program's attractiveness to teachers with different credentials and its hiring objectives. Compensation and working conditions are also important, Barnett stressed. Studies that hold those constant when examining the effects of teacher qualifications, he said, "make no sense."

Barnett suggested that research on "packages," that is, programs with particular sets of characteristics, or policy regimes, might be more useful because the features are so interactive. Certainly program effects do vary substantially, as the data in Table 4-1 show. However, data from New Jersey's Abbott Prekindergarten program show how a change in policy can

TABLE 4-1 Outcomes for Three Preschool Programs

	8 State Pre-Ks			Perry Preschool	Tulsa Pre-K	Head Start (adj)
	Avg	Lowest	Highest			
PPVT	.26	.05	.39	.75	NA	.09 (.13)
Print awareness	.97	.56	1.49	NA	.99	.25 (.34)
Math	.38	.15	.96	NA	.36	.15 (.22)

NOTE: Effect sizes are in standard deviation units, for 1 year at age 4. adj: adjusted; PPVT: Peabody Picture Vocabulary Test.
SOURCE: Barnett, 2011.

affect several child outcome measures (Frede et al., 2009). In 1999, the program raised its requirements for teachers, implemented a research-based curriculum, added master teachers, restricted class size to 15, incorporated high standards and accountability measures, and adopted a continuous improvement system. Measures of classroom quality, including the quality of the language, literacy, and mathematics environments, showed substantial improvements between the 2002–2003 and the 2008–2009 school years. The goal was overall improvement; improvement in teacher qualifications was just one part of the plan.

"We know many preschool programs are not delivering the desired results," Barnett concluded. "Inadequately prepared teachers are one likely cause, but it is not by itself the thing that's going to make a difference." Particular qualifications might bring teachers who can be highly effective, he observed, but those teachers will not necessarily be highly effective unless other things are in place. Teacher pay and working conditions, supports for teachers, the curriculum, and state and local policies have a material effect on the way teachers function in their jobs. In his view, teachers are best able to be effective when they are an integral part of a process of continual improvement. Overall, Barnett summarized his policy recommendation regarding whether teachers should have B.A. degrees in the following way: "To me when we're dealing with policy, when we're unsure, I think we have to ask 'what is the cautious thing to do?' I think moving away from programs with highly educated, well-paid teachers is an incautious thing to do given the evidence."

DISCUSSION

Workshop participants added many comments. One observed that current standards are very low, both for the individuals who enter the profession and for the level and nature of the skills and behaviors those workers are expected to have. Others highlighted the importance of effective management and well-trained professional development providers, and the need for both knowledge-oriented and practice-focused experiences in higher education teacher preparation programs. Others pointed to the need for well-defined goals, clearly agreed-on outcome measures, and timely, clear guidance about how to proceed.

Several emphasized the point that Barnett stressed—that no one single element or strategy will produce the desired quality or outcomes. However, others cautioned that evaluating combinations of factors will limit the ability to determine which of them are essential to producing the desired outcomes. One participant suggested that observational studies in addition to randomized controlled trials could be useful. Another noted that randomized experimental research focused on teacher characteristics and preparation was emerging, such as work being conducted by Susan Neuman at the University of Michigan.

Another discussion focused on the value of data-driven decision making as it relates to teacher qualifications. Although this is an important goal, several participants noted that measures of outcomes for children are very limited. "We need clearly agreed-upon outcomes that go way beyond the Peabody Picture Vocabulary Test and some of the pathetically narrow measures that we've been using in order to have the kind of robust research designs that can give us some confidence that we're on the right track," one observed. Unfortunately, applying a K–12 model for measuring outcomes is not likely to serve the early childhood context well, others noted. Social and emotional development, for example, is difficult to measure but is "an extremely important part of what we hope to stimulate with whatever kinds of care experiences children have," another noted. Furthermore, the kinds of skills, activities, and goals that are in play for infants, toddlers, and preschoolers are different, and those distinctions are not clear in the available measures.

Diversity and the Early Childhood Care and Education Workforce

Other teacher and caregiver characteristics may also influence outcomes for children, explained Ellen Frede, codirector of the National Institute for Early Education Research. She discussed the available research pertaining to two questions: (1) Is there a demographic match between caregivers[5] and the children in their care; and (2) Does a demographic match make a difference in terms of outcomes for children? The first question is not easy to answer, Frede explained. The available data pro-

---

[5] This section of the report uses the term "caregivers" as it was used in the workshop presentation.

TABLE 4-2 Demographic Matches Between Caregivers and Children in New Jersey, U.S. Census Data

2010 Census	0–5 years	All Ages	Preschool K Teachers
White alone	74.5	79.6	~ 80
Black/African American	15.2	12.9	14.2
American Indian, Alaskan Native	1.4	1	
Asian	6.3	5.7	2.6
Native Hawaiian/Pacific Islander	0.3	0.2	
Two+ races	5.3	2.2	
Hispanic	34.6	19.8	10.3
Female			97.8

SOURCE: Frede, 2011.

vide relatively little detail about caregivers' characteristics, and even less information that could be used to determine the matches between caregivers and children. Consequently, the second question is also difficult to answer, but because of its potential importance for policy it should not be overlooked, in Frede's view.

U.S. Census data provide a big-picture look, as shown in Table 4-2. Frede noted first that these data suggest it would be surprising to find a close match between caregivers and children, given that the proportion of children ages 0 to 5 who are minorities is greater than the minorities' proportion of adults in the general population.[6] The Head Start program has national enrollment data that also illuminate the issue, as shown in Table 4-3. That program has achieved a higher-than-average match rate, although the adults are more predominantly white and the children are more predominantly minority. Frede also described data for family child care in New Jersey, which shows a pattern similar to that in the Head Start data. A few studies from the 1990s looked explicitly at the matches between children and caregivers, as shown in Table 4-4, and, like the others, found lower matches for minority children.

The most significant discrepancy, she pointed out, is between His-

---

[6] Frede cautioned both that the race/ethnicity categories and the classifications for the child care and education workforce are those defined by the Census and may obscure aspects of the demographic matches.

TABLE 4-3 Demographic Matches Between Children and Caregivers, Head Start 2009–2010

2009–2010 Head Start Program Information Report		
Enrollment Statistics Report–National Level		
	Enrollment	Teaching Staff
White	39%	48%
Black/African American	31%	30%
Other race	10%	7%
Biracial or multi-racial	8%	4%
Unspecified race	6%	5%
American Indian, Alaskan Native	4%	4%
Asian	2%	2%
Native Hawaiian/Pacific Islander	1%	1%
Hispanic or Latino origin	34%	25%

SOURCE: Frede, 2011.

TABLE 4-4 Demographic Match Between Teachers and Children, Research Findings

Data Source	Euro-American	African American	Hispanic/Latino
NICHD (Burchinal and Cryer, 2003)	86%	70%	34%
CQ&O (Burchinal and Cryer, 2003)	77%	47%	42%
Multi-State Home-School Match (Barbarin et al., 2010)	90%	32%	8%

NOTE: CQ&O: Cost, Quality, and Child Outcomes in Child Care Centers Study; NICHD: National Institute of Child Health and Human Development.
SOURCE: Frede, 2011.

panic or Latino children and teachers. Demographics may make a difference if language differences impede communication and effective education. She presented some additional New Jersey data showing that providers of state-funded prekindergarten have larger percentages of bilingual teachers than do public school prekindergarten classrooms, a point discussed further below.

Why might the ethnic and racial matches between teachers and children matter? Research and theory have both suggested possible reasons, Frede explained. An older theory, based in qualitative research, was that discontinuity between home and school could be confusing to children (Silvern, 1988). It might affect teachers' attitudes toward children and also affect children's identity development. For example, children who have never had teachers of their own ethnic background might come to believe intuitively that the group from which teachers came was supposed to have more power.

Researchers have also suggested that differences in discourse patterns among ethnic groups may be important in this context. For example, Heath (1989) found that Euro-American teachers may use discourse patterns that are characterized by questions for which the adult knows the answer, while African-American parents were more likely to ask their children questions to which they actually wanted an answer. Such differences may yield misunderstanding between teachers and children.

Burchinal and Cryer (2003) have also explored the relationship between demographic matching and outcomes for children. They found that, regardless of race or ethnicity, what mattered most for outcomes were caregivers' sensitivity and the amount of stimulation they provided. These two factors predict school success across race and ethnicity. Neither a race/ethnicity match between child and caregiver nor a match of race/ethnicity and child-rearing beliefs between caregiver and parents had strong influences on outcomes for children, Frede explained. However, the researchers also stressed that there were many ways to provide sensitive and stimulating care while avoiding a disconnect with families.

Another study (Barbarin et al., 2010) also examined the effects of matches, using a slightly different description of teacher characteristics. They found, in a public prekindergarten setting, that fostering independence but providing high levels of support promoted kindergarten readiness. Even when families hold different beliefs about child rearing, teachers who follow that model improve children's readiness, though to a slightly lesser degree. In other words, Frede explained, outcomes are best if both teachers and parents use this approach, but if either one does, children will benefit.

Several studies suggest that mismatches might be a more significant issue for children who are English-language learners, Frede pointed out (Barnett et al., 2007; Durán et al., 2010; Farver et al., 2009; Gormley, 2007; Kersten et al., 2009). These studies collectively demonstrate that, in general, attending a high-quality preschool improves outcomes for English-language learners. The researchers also found that when the preschool environment uses both English and the child's home language, the children's proficiency in the home language improves, and they do not lose their progress in English.

Having a bilingual teacher is clearly a prerequisite for dual-language instruction, Frede added, but Freedson (2010) found that most dual-language children do not have a teacher who speaks their language or has specialized knowledge of this type of instruction. Moreover, Frede reported, teacher preparation programs neither routinely offer substantive coursework in linguistic or cultural diversity nor require students to learn a second language. Frede also found that bilingual teachers tend to use their (and children's) home language primarily for commands and discipline.

Frede drew several conclusions from these findings:

- The match between children and teachers in early childhood education settings with respect to race, ethnicity, and language is largely unknown but is "clearly not one-to-one";
- Perfect matching is likely not possible and, if it were, would result in de facto linguistic or racial segregation;
- What research exists suggests that demographic matches between teachers and children are not necessary for effective care and education, and that sensitive and supportive teachers are more predictive of beneficial outcomes; and
- To optimize learning for dual-language learners and increase bilingualism, more bilingual teachers need to be trained to support dual-language learning.

Frede noted that better data will be needed to shed more light on this issue. In the meantime, she believes that a few steps would make high-quality, dual-language education more widely available to children under age 5. States should require teacher preparation programs to improve bilingual education; in fact, this should be a criterion for receiving state and federal funds, she argued. She also believes that teachers should have access to professional development that fosters sensitive and stimulating interactions with children and an approach that promotes independence while providing support.

FOCUS ON WORKING CONDITIONS

The characteristics teachers and caregivers bring to the job and develop in the course of their careers are very important. The working conditions for those employed in ECCE, however, also influence the decisions prospective workers make about entering and remaining in the workforce, as well as the quality of their performance. Deborah Phillips, professor of psychology at Georgetown University, and Marcy Whitebook, senior researcher and director of the Center for the Study of Child Care Employment at the University of California, Berkeley, described research on the environmental factors that influence teachers' experiences and outcomes for children.

The Role of Stress for Children and Caregivers[7]

Phillips drew from research on the neurobiology of stress, individual differences in temperament, and child care itself to develop a portrait of the intersecting factors that affect the workforce. She briefly reviewed the evolution of research and thinking about these influences. The first wave of research on child care, she explained, focused on comparisons between children cared for at home by their mothers and those in child care. But researchers quickly realized that child care arrangements vary widely and began looking for the ingredients that make it effective.

The next phase of research explored ecological models. Researchers attempted to control for the impacts of home environments and parenting, to control for selection bias in their study samples (i.e., unobserved factors that may influence the type of children served by different child care settings), and to focus not only on the setting for child development, but also on the setting for adult workers. More recent work examines interactions between child care and parenting and the relationships between parents and caregivers. Current work is also focusing on the theory that quality in child care is not necessarily linear, and that certain thresholds may need to be reached before the positive benefits of child care can be demonstrated.

At the same time, advances in research on child development—and especially early brain development—and on the neurobiology of stress have shed light on the critical role played by caregivers. The developing brain, Phillips explained, is designed to "greedily recruit from the environments and experiences that surround it as they shape its emerging architecture and neurochemistry." Early experiences "literally mold the brain," but it will recruit both supportive and damaging experiences. A critical element in this process is the development of the structure that manages the brain's and body's response to stress (the hypothalamic-pituitary-adrenal [HPA] axis). This system produces cortisol, a steroid hormone that plays a critical role in adaptation to stressful stimuli. Researchers have found that regular and sustained activation of this system in animals early in life is associated with increased fearfulness and impairment of the capacity to regulate responses (Gunnar, 2008; NSCDC, 2005). In particular, these animals' responses to novelty, struggles for dominance, and reactions to social threats are affected.

Efforts to understand the circumstances under which activation of the HPA system has adaptive or non-adaptive effects have led to the development of a three-part classification of stress, Phillips explained: positive stress, tolerable stress, and toxic stress (NSCDC, 2005). Positive stress is

---

[7] This section of the report uses the term "caregivers" as it was used in the workshop presentation.

mild and temporary, and promotes the developing capacity to respond to the inevitable stress of life. Tolerable stress is more enduring and intense, but does not compromise the developing HPA system, often because of the buffering presence of a dependable and responsive adult. Toxic stress includes stress in the absence of protective factors (e.g., a supportive adult) or severe abuse, neglect, or prolonged maternal depression that deprives the child of the secure presence of a loving adult.

Although every developing child would be affected by toxic stress, Phillips explained, some are more vulnerable than others. Researchers believe that children's innate temperaments can affect their capacity to regulate their stress response systems—and some are characterized by "negative reactivity" (Martin and Fox, 2008; Rothbart et al., 2006). Different temperaments can be detected in babies as young as age 4 months. When they are presented with intense stimuli, such as loud noises, busy pictures, and multiple people, some "freak out—they arch their backs and cry"; they are clearly miserable. Babies at the other end of the spectrum may thrive on the same level of stimulation. As they grow, a share of the infants with highly negative reactions remains easily stressed and exhibits high anxiety and high cortisol levels in stressful social situations.

These children, Phillips explained, are particularly sensitive to their contexts, including variations in the quality of the care they experience in their first months and years. When these children do not receive dependable, sensitive care, they tend to display one of two behavioral profiles: fearful, anxious retreat from stressful situations, or aggression and lack of behavioral control. When they do receive dependable, sensitive care, however, they are usually able to develop well-calibrated stress response systems.

This work, Phillips noted, has focused researchers' thinking about the conditions under which child care may compromise development, and the conditions under which children thrive in child care. This perspective, she added, "really ups the ante on how we think about the adults who are caring for young children. What responsibilities are we really placing in their hands? It goes way beyond … dressing, feeding, bathing, and overseeing play." Evidence has long been clear that child care varies widely in quality and that its quality matters a lot to children's outcomes, she noted. Now, new data indicate that poor-quality child care appears to be a highly stressful environment for a particular group of children. They display rising levels of cortisol over the course of the day in child care that they do not exhibit at home—whereas the normal pattern is for cortisol levels to be highest at the start of the day and to drop in the course of the day.

Emerging evidence indicates that this circumstance may profoundly affect these children's development. Inhibited, fearful, socially reticent children seem to be the most vulnerable, especially at ages 2 and 3 (Phillips et al., 2011). "These are children who are on the periphery of the action a lot of the time," she explained. "They are seen watching rather than participating in play and social activities, but they're not watching happily. They are feeling left out. They are really anxious. They're self-soothing. They're clinging to adults. It's really painful to observe these children." Studies are beginning to show that poor-quality care is associated with a higher incidence of stress responses in children, whether in center- or home-based programs (Phillips et al., 2011). The elevated cortisol has also been associated with increased frequency of infections and lower antibody levels.

What is still missing is a clear way to determine the threshold at which child care moves from stressful to beneficial. Intrusive, overcontrolling care, she added, appears to have a negative influence, while warm, sensitive care has a positive effect. Emerging research suggests specifically that a secure attachment between the child and his or her lead teacher seems to protect against the rising cortisol levels (Badanes et al., 2011; Gunnar et al., 2011). Existing measures of child care quality are not bad, Phillips observed, but they are "missing something really important" because they do not capture this aspect of care. Another area of concern is the mental and emotional state of the caregivers and teachers themselves, Phillips explained. Some research has shown that 16 percent of family child care providers and 22 percent of center teachers have scores above the threshold for genuine depression (Whitebook et al., 2004). In both settings, those who care for low-income children have the highest rates of depression. Some have reported links between caregiver depression and intrusive, overcontrolling care that has a negative effect. Those who care for children on their own are most vulnerable to depression that can interfere with the quality of care. The emerging evidence suggests that, like children, some caregivers exhibit rising cortisol levels in the course of the day, and this effect is negatively associated with child well-being.

This body of work, in Phillips' view, makes it clear that caregivers need to know how to help children navigate and manage peer interaction and how to help them develop the self-regulatory and executive functioning skills that underlie both social competence and cognitive and language development. Caregivers need to be perceptive about and sensitive to individual differences among children. Caregivers with these characteristics and skills are particularly important for children with any kind of vulnerability related to temperament or special needs or poverty. Phillips also emphasized that child care for all children must be understood as an intervention—one that will affect their developmental trajectories, "either in an adaptive or a compromised direction."

Stability and Stress

Whitebook presented data on turnover and other aspects of the workplace that can contribute to teacher and caregiver well-being and quality. Child care environments vary tremendously, she observed. Worker turnover, stress, and skill levels are intertwined, and these interactions are important to center quality (she noted that most of the research in this area focuses on centers rather than home-based care).

Job turnover can be positive, Whitebook noted, when it means that staff who are not very effective are leaving the field, or that individuals are leaving jobs that do not reward their investment in education and professional development. Conversely, stability is not a positive sign when workers stay because they believe they have no other opportunities, receive no encouragement to improve, or do not experience consequences for failure to improve. In any case, job turnover in child care is very high, as the right-hand column in Table 4-5 shows. Some evidence suggests it is highest for those who work with infants and toddlers, who are also the most vulnerable to the consequences of turnover. For example, a study of child care workers in California showed that turnover was 29 percent in centers that serve infants and toddlers as well as older children, and 20 percent for those that serve only older children (Whitebook et al., 2006). Turnover was highest in centers that serve children in subsidized programs. Turnover in family child care has been less well researched, but one Illinois study found a rate of 25 percent turnover over a 15-month period for licensed family providers (Fowler et al., 2008). Another California study found that among providers who were receiving a subsidy to care for children whose mothers had just stopped receiving welfare benefits, 43 percent left in the course of a year (Whitebook et al., 2003).

Numerous factors may influence turnover in any occupation, Whitebook explained. Poor compensation, poor hiring decisions, and poor working conditions are the most frequent causes. In the early childhood context, wages appear to be an especially significant factor. Table

TABLE 4-5 Wages and Stability

Occupation	Mean Hourly Wage	Turnover Rate
Registered nurses	$31.99	5%
K–8 teachers	$30.60	10%
Social workers	$24.26	10%
Preschool teachers	$13.20	15%
Home health aides/nurse's aides	$10.39	18%
Child care workers	$10.07	29%
Food counter workers	$ 9.13	42%

SOURCE: Whitebook, 2011; Based on U.S. Department of Labor, Bureau of Labor Statistics, 2009.

4-5 also shows the hourly wages for child care workers and several other occupations, and demonstrates an inverse relationship between salary and turnover rate. Despite the fact that unemployment is currently very high and states and other jurisdictions are struggling with serious budget shortfalls, Whitebook stressed, relative compensation for child care workers is still important. The Department of Defense, she noted, has demonstrated that it was possible to sharply reduce turnover in the military child care system without passing on the labor costs to parents. Faced with a turnover rate of 48 percent in 1989, the Department of Defense instituted a new pay and training plan. They made pay for child care jobs commensurate with that for other jobs with similar requirements for education and training. The turnover rate was reduced to 24 percent by 1993 (Campbell et al., 2000).

Children experience turnover in their teachers and caregivers as loss, Whitebook explained, and it affects the quality of their care. A 1989 study (Whitebook et al., 1990) showed, for example, that children in centers with low quality and high turnover have poorer language and social development. Other work (Whitebook et al., 2001, 2004) showed that centers that were able to improve their ECERS scores, gain accreditation, and sustain those improvements were also those that had the lowest turnover and paid the highest wages. She added that directors and teachers "talk about turnovers as the time sponge, the energy drain, or the plague, depending on how bad it is." Finding a replacement for the worker who has left may take 3 to 6 weeks. Children may need to be regrouped, and "conversation with children stops because everybody is just trying to keep their heads above water." Because of pressure to fill the position quickly and meet ratio requirements, directors may end up hiring people who are less skilled (the "warm body" syndrome), and quality declines. Often the result is additional turnover, as well as stress for teachers, caregivers, parents, and directors. Turnover among directors is also a problem, which can both exacerbate and be exacerbated by staff turnover.

Among caregivers who leave child care jobs, Whitebook noted, data show that about 42 percent move to other centers, 8 percent move to resource and referral agencies, 7 percent move to K–12 education, and 21 percent leave the field altogether (Whitebook et al., 2001). A survey of people working in resource and referral agencies found that about 50 percent had a background working in child care—and that two-thirds of those people said they have left direct child care because of the pay (Whitebook et al., 2010).

Even though having any job in a time of high unemployment is better than none, working for very low wages is nevertheless stressful. One study (Whitebook et al., 2011) has shown that only 44 percent of child care workers would be able to support themselves and their families on their own wages alone. Only about a third of child care workers have employer-paid benefits or paid sick leave. These conditions are stressful, and, as Phillips discussed, stress and depression among caregivers can have negative effects on children. Whitebook added that working with stressed and depressed colleagues can be stressful in itself and undermine the professional culture in a center.

In general, she observed, the turnover problem is an aspect of the broader challenge of ensuring that child care and education programs are staffed by people who have the appropriate skills (e.g., dual-language training, special education experience), the credentials, and the social support necessary. The work environment is a critical ingredient in quality child care, she believes, but most states use quality rating and improvement systems that do not really address what is necessary to create a positive work environment. A few states (Colorado, Illinois, and New Mexico) have begun to focus on workplace quality, but most have not yet done so, Whitebook and colleagues found (Austin et al., 2011). Although further research will be needed to support firm conclusions, Whitebook and her colleagues identified several working conditions that are likely to be important:

- A workplace that is a learning environment in which workers have the opportunity to reflect on and discuss their work;
- A workplace in which people are empowered to make changes as they learn new strategies and skills;
- The resources necessary for adult well-being, such as mental health referrals for workers who are having problems or paid leave for illness; and
- Adequate financial rewards.

The well-being of the adults in early childhood settings—their living and working conditions—are not a distraction from the needs of children, Whitebook added, but rather the cornerstone of children's environment, and thus an essential determinant of how well children are going to do.

DISCUSSION

Participants identified additional workforce issues that also merit further investigation. One described a "disconnect" between (1) what researchers have learned about children's development and the care they need, and (2) the way the field conceptualizes the skills the workforce needs and approaches recruitment. The low status the occupation currently has, together with the low wages, is likely to continue to limit its appeal to academically successful college graduates. Others worried that as expectations for child care and education are raised, the workforce who can deliver that level of competence is just not available. The workforce needs a range of financial as well as non-monetary supports if quality is to improve, they suggested.

5

Building the Workforce and the Profession

D efining and describing the people who comprise the early childhood care and education (ECCE) workforce is an incomplete task without considering the context that helps to shape some of their characteristics. The professional development, compensation, career opportunities, recognition, and working conditions of the ECCE workforce provide some of these important contextual elements. They influence who enters and stays in the workforce, as well as the quality and effectiveness of their services for children and families. These contextual elements are shaped by market forces, as well as by local, state, and federal policies.

Joan Lombardi, deputy assistant secretary and interdepartmental liaison for early childhood development at the Administration for Children and Families of the U.S. Department of Health and Human Services, provided her views on the policy context of the ECCE workforce. Although she noted the substantial improvements that states and federal programs have made in addressing early learning standards and quality rating and improvement systems, she expressed her view that efforts targeting the workforce deserve to be a much greater priority for policy makers. She emphasized the point that innovative strategies are needed to reach those who provide care and education in homes, both in family child care settings as well as in the homes of the large numbers of family, friends, and neighbors who provide child care, regardless of their status as members of the ECCE profession.

Lombardi described her concern that the ECCE field needs—but may not currently have—a workforce that is adequately prepared to take on the challenges of using today's evidence-based practices. A particular challenge is the expectations we are putting on teachers in all early childhood programs without the adequate preparation, support, and compensation they need. She expressed her concern that "in our efforts to align everything, we are placing expectations on a completely under-resourced child care system. That is a problem," particularly given the challenging working conditions of much of the workforce.

She highlighted several federal initiatives to address the needs of a broad range of the ECCE workforce, including Head Start's National Center for Teaching and Learning, programs to support home-based providers, and the expansion of mentoring programs for teachers. She also noted her optimism in seeing the energy, creativity, and intentionality of young teachers, including those from Teach for America and so many other new teachers, who are dedicating their work to young children. Lombardi's recent experiences engaging directly with teachers focused her attention on the challenges ahead, the distance still to go to achieve desired outcomes for the workforce, and the promise of new strategies.

The final session of the workshop was dedicated to exploring the context of the ECCE workforce, including its challenges and promising efforts to address them. Considering how to build ECCE as a "profession" was an important theme explored in this session. A perspective from health care offered a useful example of how a profession (e.g., nursing) can have a shared identity among individuals who work in a diverse range of settings, improve standards and requirements for entry, and foster means for continuing improvement. Presenters also explored perspectives on the career pathways, training and education, and working conditions that affect this workforce. Discussion highlighted possible steps for the future to support the workforce and better serve the children and families whose lives they touch.

LEARNING FROM THE HEALTH CARE EXPERIENCE

Other fields have struggled with many of the same issues that face the ECCE workforce and the policy makers and others who hope to strengthen it. Catherine Dower, associate director of research at the Center for the Health Professions at the University of California, San Francisco, drew some comparisons with health care and suggested a template for evaluating emerging professions.

Dower reported that although we spend more money on health care than any other nation, and more than 11 million people work in health care in the United States, we rank below virtually all other industrialized countries on adverse health-related measures, such as deaths from medical errors, preventable deaths, and contracting infections in hospitals. Health care workers are part of both the problem and the solution, Dower suggested.

All professions constantly evolve, in response to changes in technology, consumer demands, and demographic changes, and new professions emerge as well. Dower and colleagues (2001) developed a template to evaluate new and emerging health care professions, such as acupuncture, naturopathic medicine, and homeopathic medicine. This tool has since been used in many contexts because it provides a standard way to identify benchmarks to gauge progress relative to other fields, and to calibrate expectations related to cost, access, choice, quality, and culturally appropriate care or service. Dower explained that the tool is designed for use by consumers as well as professionals and researchers.

The model is not quantitative, she added. It does not impose time lines or set numeric goals. Rather, it is a subjective way of identifying key issues and questions. The model organizes the questions into five categories: (1) defining and describing the profession; (2) safety and efficacy issues; (3) government and private-sector recognition; (4) education and training; and (5) proactive practice model and viability of profession.

1. *Defining and describing the profession.* What services are offered? Is there consensus among the members of the workgroup on how to define the profession? The professions that have been most successful are those that have been able to develop a shared definition, Dower noted. It is also important to describe the areas of overlap with other professions, to consider the value of what the particular profession adds, what distinguishes it from others, and how it developed. Data are important as well—the size of the workforce, its demographics, and its growth trends. Most important is to ask whether the workforce is large enough and has the right skills to meet the needs of the population it serves.

2. *Safety and efficacy issues.* Dower stressed that these are separate issues, though they are treated together. Safety issues concern the potential of risk or harm to the client or consumer, and are the reasons why professions are licensed by states. Many professions, she noted, seek regulation both as protection and as a signal of their value, and are thus compelled to make arguments to the legislature about the ways in which their practitioners could harm the public without adequate regulation. Consumers are most concerned with efficacy, and professions need an agenda for research to expand their understanding of what works and what is most important in their practice, as well as a means of disseminating the findings.

3. *Government and private-sector recognition.* Professions need to consider the ways third parties view their work and their practitioners, and have strategies for seeking recognition for their work. In addition to regulation, structures for payment—including insurance, financing, and third-party reimbursement—play important roles. Professions also need to understand who is seeking their services, why, and how clients or consumers locate practitioners. Private-sector (non-government) certification is important in this context because it provides a way to signal to potential consumers that a practitioner meets professional standards. The development of such standards should be based on a job analysis, and the certification should be based on some type of assessment.

4. *Education and training.* Most professions do have some college-based or vocational school-based preparation as well as practice-based training. Some professions have an apprenticeship track, as well. Some lay and direct-entry professional midwives, for example, have an apprenticeship track that is recognized, and also have national certification. One important element for professions to consider is how well their education system prepares candidates for accreditation, and what continuing education is available. The education and training must also prepare those who will do research on the profession and serve as faculty for future professionals.

5. *Proactive practice model and viability of profession.* What the profession is currently doing and can do in the future to develop new and better ways to provide their services is a critical question for the ECCE field. Dower placed special emphasis on this element, noting that health care and service industries are changing quickly because of technology, financing issues, and demographic changes both within the workforce and within the populations they serve. Existing and emerging fields have taken different pathways in this climate of rapid change, but several factors are widely shared. The most important ingredient in keeping them viable, she added, is leadership, and leaders within the 200-plus recognized health professions have looked to education, certification, and licensure tools to help them gain public recognition and stay current.

Public understanding is important, even though it may seem like an extraneous factor, Dower added. Most medical fields are viewed as necessities, but a few—such as branches of alternative medicine—are viewed as options. From an outside perspective, ECCE often seems to be in that category as well. Box 5-1 presents six questions to guide thinking about how a profession can be proactive.

Dower closed with two key points. First, a profession's ability to understand and adapt to change is an indication of its viability. Perhaps most important in this regard is for the members and leaders of the profession to have both sufficient information to understand what needs to be changed and sufficient freedom and resources to try new approaches. Data and research that analyzes the data's meaning, a leadership infrastructure, and individuals who will persist in pushing for change are all key ingredients. Second, a profession's role in leading positive change is an indication of its strength in defining and improving care. She stressed her sense that policy makers and the public do not understand the ECCE field well. A public relations effort that builds understanding of the vital responsibility these workers assume, the powerful benefits they can bring to children and families, and the challenges and obstacles that affect their work could be a valuable contribution. When this template is applied to the ECCE workforce, gaps that need further attention can be identified.

CAREER PATHWAYS FOR WORKERS

Marcy Whitebook, senior researcher and director of the Center for the Study of Child Care Employment at the University of California, Berkeley, presented an overview of the interrelated contextual challenges facing today's ECCE workforce. Differences among caregivers and teachers—in their purpose and goals, the care they provide, and their education and training—are vast and often reinforced by regulation and funding streams, she noted. Some members of the workforce consider themselves to be professionals, but others do not. Those in the K–12 system will have earned certification before entering the classroom. However, many who work in ECCE settings rarely face such certification requirements to enter the field. These individuals may have little more than cardiopulmonary resuscitation training while working, and often pursue job-related training or education only after they have already been working with young children for a significant period of time. Entry requirements for ECCE jobs vary widely ranging from "16 or older and breathing" to a master's degree and certification. As Whitebook stated, "We haven't even articulated what the expectations and competencies are for people in all sorts of different roles," a problem which complicates setting entry requirements to the field and assuring consumers of a standard of competence.

Members of K–3 settings, she added, have a clear expectation that teachers' knowledge and skills will develop over time. Support programs for new teachers, mentoring, professional development, and paid planning time are standard practices in that context. The pathway to leader-

---

BOX 5-1
Questions to Guide a Proactive Practice Model

Are there practice guidelines? Dower noted that although she is critical of medicine on many points, the field has been serious about developing standards and guidelines so that practitioners are working toward the same goals, and also continually working to identify and rectify weaknesses. She particularly noted the contribution of the Institute for Health Care Improvement, which developed the 100,000 Lives Campaign in response to the Institute of Medicine report (IOM, 1999) on medical errors. This campaign began with easy changes every hospital can make, such as improved cleaning of the site of an IV (intravenous) needle, which can immediately reduce infection rates. The Institute for Health Care Improvement has since increased both the target in lives to be saved and the number of key practices. The campaign is important in part because these are all practices that staff already know how to do, yet improving adherence to them is "changing the face of medicine."

Are there interprofessional teams? The problem of "fiefdoms" that may duplicate one another's efforts or work at cross-purposes may be at its worst in medicine, Dower suggested, but some promising developments are addressing the problem. For example, medical doctors, nurse practitioners, and physician assistants have increased their collaboration, which benefits all three. Nurse practitioners and physician assistants are trained to do much of the routine care in primary and specialty practices, and when they are able to do so, the medical doctor can focus on complex situations where expert judgment is needed. Such models are effective both clinically and financially, she added.

Are clients satisfied and how is that measured? Understanding what clients, patients, and consumers think about the care being provided is critical, Dower explained, and this information can be obtained in a variety of ways. Practitioners are increasingly asking patients for feedback, though Dower noted that these data need to be collected systematically and tracked so that trends can be identified. Nurses, she added, have been particularly diligent about conducting national and

---

ship roles is also relatively clearly defined in the K–3 context, at least by comparison with other early education settings. Demographic differences in the profiles of workers in the various settings that provide care and education also reflect status differences, as some California data suggest. In that state, 26 percent of K–12 teachers, 47 percent of teachers in ECCE centers, and 58 percent of licensed providers are non-white (while 70 percent of children they care for are non-white). As she had previously described, the K–12 teachers earn the most and have the lowest rates of turnover, and a greater percentage of them are male.

From the point of view of young people considering career path-

other surveys. They point with pride to their status as the most trusted profession in the United States, according to the Gallup Poll, which conducts an annual survey of the public to rank professions for their honesty and ethical standards.

Is the field innovative? Nurses have also set an excellent example here, Dower noted. Through the Integrated Nurse Leadership Program in California, for example, nurses were given the authority to develop new ways to reduce infection rates and mistakes in hospitals. They developed new techniques and systems and were able to make significant improvements in both areas. Technology has also exceeded expectations as a feasible option for allowing care to be delivered remotely, Dower noted, and has provided more avenues for innovation.

Are practitioners and care or service accessible? Being truly accessible, Dower explained, begins with attention to geographic, language, and financial issues. Professionals need to be available and practicing in the neighborhoods where people live. Addressing this problem requires data on where practitioners are located and the languages they speak (and how well). The financial issues are complex in the current political environment, but working to make affordable care available is nonetheless a key responsibility of these professions.

Are there professional and advocacy groups to advance the profession? These groups take the lead in both articulating and pursuing goals for the profession and are its most public face. A leadership structure is necessary for those things to happen, however, and Dower noted how frequently the leadership is fractured in medicine and other fields. She looked again to nursing as an example of how that problem can be addressed. Each state regulates nurse practitioners differently, and wide variation exists in the scope of practice. As a result, nurse practitioners cannot easily move from state to state—"it's almost not the same profession," she noted, "so it's a big problem." For many years nursing groups were in conflict, but a group of leading nursing organizations has developed a consensus model that they hope can rectify the situation. Dower pointed to models for this approach in other professions as well (Goffin, 2009).

ways, she suggested, the most attractive pathway is clearly the K–12 job. Whitebook shared the words of one director:

> I see these young girls starting out in the early childhood teaching field today and I want to say, "Do you realize what you're doing? You're spending a lot of time getting into a field that's not going to offer you anything in the long term." And I really hate to say that, because teachers are needed.

What is needed, in Whitebook's view, is a system that works well for workers with varying backgrounds and aspirations, whether they embark on the path having little more than a high school diploma, having taken early childhood classes at a community college, or having achieved a bachelor's degree (B.A.) or higher. As it is now, the system is difficult to navigate and few sources of information and support for either young people or more experienced workers looking for ways to advance exist to help them make decisions about employment and education. For example, courses offered at the community college may or may not help teachers and caregivers in their jobs, may not be of high quality, and may not help them earn more or advance. Counseling and peer support, as well as scholarships and financial aid, are important supports. Many prospective and current teachers and caregivers also need flexible school and work schedules to continue their education, as well as tutoring and computer supports (Whitebook et al., 2011).

A variety of efforts to address these challenges is under way, Whitebook noted. Several states have developed career ladders for early childhood workers that strengthen their higher education capacity and other training options. Improving wages poses a more difficult challenge in the current economic environment—and indeed at any time—but it is a critical contribution, she added. Efforts to improve data collection and to develop more standard protocols so that states can more easily share data are under way. These efforts may help states provide more consistent opportunities for workers. Whitebook concluded that no single tool will improve what she described as the infrastructure of the ECCE workforce. She stressed the importance and interrelatedness of preparation, support for ongoing learning, and rewards. "If we just build one piece then it's not going to be an efficient system."

EDUCATION AND TRAINING

Education and training are critical components to having an ECCE workforce that is able to meet the needs of children and families. Pamela Winton, senior scientist and director of outreach at the Frank Porter Graham Child Development Institute at the University of North Carolina at Chapel Hill, provided an overview of the current system and the issues it presents. She focused her presentation on six questions developed by the workshop planning committee:

1. What do we know about the education and training of the early care and education workforce?
2. How does the early childhood field recognize the credibility of education and training programs?
3. How do individuals demonstrate their knowledge and skills in conjunction with education and training programs, and how does that relate to certification?

4. Are education and training opportunities standardized at the state, regional, or local levels?
5. To what extent are professional development providers certified, expected to demonstrate specific knowledge and skills, and supported in their own development?
6. Are education and training integrated across key sectors (child care, Head Start, public prekindergarten, early intervention) or organized separately within individual sectors?

She concluded her presentation by summarizing her views and providing a set of recommendations.

1. What do we know about the education and training of the early care and education workforce?

First, she noted, information about workforce participation in education and training is not neatly organized or easy to find. One challenge relates to the definition of these terms. One might think that education is what happens before individuals enter the field and training is the additional education they receive while on the job. In practice, however, individuals take so many pathways to employment, degrees, and certification that clear, agreed-on definitions are difficult, making it hard to interpret the existing data, she explained (Maxwell et al., 2006). The field also lacks data collection systems that adequately document the education and training of ECCE workers. Some states have training registries, often limited to one sector (e.g., child care), but national data on workforce participation in education and training or on those who provide education and training experiences do not exist.

Winton uses the inclusive term "professional development" as defined by the National Professional Development Center on Inclusion, an organization devoted to assisting states in improving professional development for early childhood educators (Buysse et al., 2009; NPDCI, 2008)[1]:

> Professional development is facilitated teaching and learning experiences that are transactional and designed to support the acquisition of professional knowledge, skills, and dispositions as well as the application of this knowledge in practice. (NPDCI, 2008, p. 3)

This definition includes both preservice education and subsequent training on the theory that the nature of the education is more important than when or where it takes place. The key aspects of professional development to be assessed would be the characteristics and contexts of the

---

[1] See http://community.fpg.unc.edu/ for more information.

learners (the "who"), the content imparted (the "what"), and the way in which the learning experience is organized and presented (the "how").

2. How does the early childhood field recognize the credibility of education and training programs?

Not only are few data available for enumerating and evaluating professional development, but also numerous sectors exist within the field of ECCE (e.g., child care, Head Start, public prekindergarten, early intervention, preschool disabilities, family support, and so on) with funding and authority for providing early childhood professional development. These points may partly account for the difficulty the field has had in settling on professional standards, Winton observed, adding that the field has too many sets of standards and means of accreditation. Although each may have value, a lack of integration leads to numerous gaps and duplications.[2] The standards are mostly voluntary and may not be as useful as they could be because they do not fully reflect emerging research in developmental and educational science and changing demographics in the field, for example.

Winton described a number of promising efforts. The National Association for the Education of Young Children (NAEYC) and the Division for Early Childhood of the Council for Exceptional Children (DEC/CEC) have begun to align their standards, and Zero to Three, a nonprofit group focused on the welfare of infants and toddlers, is defining the competencies needed by people across sectors who work with very young children, and structuring professional development goals that align with them (Gebhard et al., 2010).

3. How do individuals demonstrate their knowledge and skills in conjunction with education and training programs, and how does that relate to certification?

The way in which individuals can learn and demonstrate the knowledge and skills they have gained from education and training is another question mark for the field, Winton observed. Research linking practitioners' practice-based knowledge and their use of evidence-based practices to improve outcomes for children and families holds promise as a way of structuring professional development and evaluation. Unfortu-

---

[2] Winton noted that organizations that have standards for early childhood educators include NAEYC, the Teacher Education Accreditation Council, National Council for Accreditation of Teacher Education, National Board for Professional Teaching Standards, Child Development Association, and Council for Exceptional Children.

nately, Winton noted, most professional development still places the most emphasis on induction, general compliance, and general knowledge, and relatively little on research-based practices (Lambert et al., 2010).

In Winton's view, systematically integrating existing standards across early childhood sectors and making explicit links to practices will be important. The CONNECT Project (the Center to Mobilize Early Childhood Knowledge) is addressing this need by designing instructional modules for early childhood faculty and professional development providers that are focused on research-based practices drawn from the professional and program standards of the NAEYC, DEC/CEC, and Head Start. The modules are designed to develop teachers' capacity to use multiple sources of evidence in making decisions about their practice. Another promising example is the "My Teaching Partner" program, a professional development component of the Classroom Assessment Scoring System (CLASS) (Pianta et al., 2005), a widely used observational measure of classroom quality.

4. Are education and training opportunities standardized at the state, regional, or local levels?

Ideally, education and training opportunities would be standardized at the state, national, and local levels. However, Winton suggested that the field should be able to answer "What do we know about effective professional development that we would want to standardize?" Small-scale programs have been recognized as effective, but bringing them to scale remains a challenge. Although much has been written about what constitutes effective professional development, she noted, "there is only a tiny, slim body of research that demonstrates the causal connection among early childhood professional development, research-based practices, and child and family outcomes." That is true in the K–12 context (Wei et al., 2009) and in the context of special education (Goe and Coggshall, 2007) as well, she added, noting that "we just don't have the rigorous studies."

Unfortunately, she noted, this means that when policy makers ask how professional development dollars should be invested, the answer has to be "it's complicated." The answer depends on the "who" (who are the learners and who is available to implement the professional development?), the "what" (what do the learners need to know and be able to do?), and the infrastructure support for change (factors such as access, outreach, and resources).

At this stage, Winton explained that the research community has developed several themes to guide effective professional development approaches:

- Focus on research-based practices rather than general knowledge;
- Include learning opportunities that are of sufficient duration and intensity and that address the need for guided practice and corrective feedback;
- Provide regular opportunities for collaborative problem solving and shared inquiry and learning;
- Connect the content and methods of professional development with program standards, curriculums, and assessments used in practice; and
- Determine how to establish teacher/caregiver proficiency for specific early care and education practices.

Given the relatively general guidance available from research, Winton stressed that "one size does not fit all." Being responsive to practical needs in particular circumstances is important. For example, if a new regulation has been imposed, workers might benefit from a one-time workshop or webinar to build awareness, even though that model does not fit the vision she had just described. Nevertheless, the intensive, sustained approaches hold the most promise for building the kind of skilled workforce described throughout the workshop as most effective.

Moreover, she suggested that developing operational definitions and identifying essential features of consultation, coaching, and mentoring should happen before spending freely on these strategies. Given cost constraints, she added, the possibilities for using technology to deliver some forms of professional development must be carefully explored. For example, many faculty report significant difficulty in locating high-quality settings for students to conduct the practical component of their training. At the same time, administrators and supervisors complain about recent graduates who have no idea how to work with ethnically and linguistically diverse children. Video demonstrations of exemplary practices offer a means of bridging logistical gaps for programs.

5. To what extent are professional development providers certified, expected to demonstrate specific knowledge and skills, and supported in their own development?

Winton raised other questions about the standards for those who deliver professional development—how they are evaluated and the nature of the pipeline that prepares the faculty and trainers. This area is very undeveloped, she explained. Some state training registries list professional development providers, but, in general, few people are thinking about this issue. Data are not adequate to describe the knowledge, skills, and practices of those who are delivering education and training (Hyson et al., in press). A few programs support faculty development, she noted, including CONNECT, ResearchConnections, and the U.S. Department of Education, Office of Special Education Programs, which runs a competitive grant program for innovations in preparation programs and leadership development.

6. Are education and training integrated across key sectors (child care, Head Start, public prekindergarten, early intervention) or organized separately within individual sectors?

Winton observed that one of the most pressing needs in addressing the workforce challenges is for all involved in the ECCE enterprise to join forces across sectors, especially in lean budgetary times. Existing early childhood systems are not well integrated. Multiple professional development initiatives are ongoing across child care, Head Start, public prekindergarten, preschool disabilities, and early intervention programs, each with different funding streams, missions, and standards (Buysse et al., 2009; Winton et al., 2008). "Whether we call it a profession, a workforce, a sector, or an industry," she added, "there has got to be a way to put it all together or we are going to be in trouble." The challenge is that people working in these fields, with good intentions, tend to work in silos, or "fiefdoms." They are going to have to "give up unilateral control of money, autonomy, and authority" if they are to break down the boundaries that constrain integration, she noted.

Efforts at the state level hold some promise in this respect. Many state-level early childhood agencies have increased their emphasis on building systems that function across sectors, and have included professional development in their thinking, she observed. Many national technical assistance projects funded by the U.S. Department of Health and Human Services and the U.S. Department of Education are working on sharing tools and building partnerships through the National Early Childhood Technical Assistance Consortium.

In summary, Winton identified four primary challenges related to the professional development of the ECCE field: (1) lack of a clear definition of professional development; (2) existence of many varied national standards; (3) lack of attention to the quality of professional development, including the use of evidence-based practices and the providers of professional development; and (4) the voluntary and fragmented nature of existing efforts to improve the quality of professional development in ECCE. She closed with four recommendations for improving professional development. Leaders representing the major early childhood sectors should work together to accomplish the following goals:

- Develop a shared definition of key terms related to professional development;
- Develop a uniform certification/licensure program based on national standards and related core competencies that are linked to research-based practices;
- Develop expectations and supports for the providers of professional development; and
- Invest in rigorous experimental investigations of professional development interventions.

PANEL DISCUSSION ON EDUCATION AND TRAINING

A panel of discussants pursued several themes from this presentation. Tammy Mann, executive director of the Frederick D. Patterson Research Institute of the United Negro College Fund, focused on the importance of building diversity in the workforce, and incorporating that perspective into education and training. She noted that postsecondary institutions differ markedly in the rates at which they graduate young people with diverse backgrounds, with 2-year institutions having the greatest success. Historically black 4-year colleges and universities, she added, graduate (proportionally) the greatest number of individuals who are diverse and are interested in early education, as well as the greatest number of men interested in this female-dominated field.

Another concern for Mann was the general lack of preparedness of young people entering postsecondary education, which ultimately influences the readiness of early childhood workers. Deficiencies in academic skills and in social, emotional, and financial skills, as well as in the willingness to persist and succeed, impede young people's progress, she suggested. These issues affect the pipeline for early childhood workers, and she advocated devoting resources to address this problem.

Sharon Ramey, professor and distinguished Carilion Research Scholar at Virginia Polytechnic Institute and State University, also focused on basic qualifications for work in ECCE. Other fields have basic prerequisites: pilots must meet requirements for vision and hearing, and medical students are screened for mental health problems, for example. These workers need not only good mental and physical health, but also resistance to disease, health care coverage (so they can return to work quickly if they are ill or injured), physical stamina, energy, empathy, and patience. They also need to know health and safety practices for children of different ages, and to understand social and emotional development. They need to understand how children communicate and learn, and how to communicate with families. They probably also need "exceptional open-mindedness," she added, because in this field they are likely to be called on repeatedly to change their practice. They also need pride in their work and a commitment to its importance. They need to understand the high stakes associated with their work and be prepared to be held accountable for it.

Martha Zaslow, director of the Office for Policy and Communications at the Society for Research on Child Development and senior scientist at Child Trends, reminded the group of the progress made both in higher education and in the universe of training for workers. The National Council for Accreditation of Teacher Education and NAEYC accreditation programs for higher education are national attempts to ensure quality, she noted. The difficulty is that only a fraction of programs apply and about 25 percent are asked to reapply each year because they do not meet the criteria. Programs that face recurring difficulties present an important warning sign, and some programs are even asked not to proceed with their applications. Most such programs, she explained, are not adequately focused on early childhood. Zaslow recommended further study of whether the graduates of these programs actually engage in observably different practices, as well as whether differences exist in the populations that select and enroll in different programs.

Zaslow also noted national efforts to provide quality markers for training, including individual credentialing, program accreditation, and identification of qualified professional development providers. Research is needed here as well, but she cautioned that, for example, an "explosion" of research on coaching has occurred without producing a coherent description of the elements that make coaching successful.

RECOGNITION OF THE WORKFORCE

Sue Russell, president of the Child Care Services Association, examined several factors that affect the quality of the workforce and the recognition it receives. She drew on her experience working in North Carolina and working with other states across the country, and her themes reflected much of the workshop discussion, as well. First, the workforce is largely composed of women working for low wages and few benefits. Most have taken a few college courses. A surprising number were first-generation college students, and many struggle with mathematics and literacy requirements as they begin their college education. This population is more racially and ethnically diverse than the typical K–12 teacher population. A large proportion of this workforce would like to earn more credentials and degrees, but it is not easy for them to do so, she added. They need comprehensive supports to progress, and they deserve to see their compensation increase as they make educational progress, she argued.

The challenge, in Russell's view, is to make sustainable improvements in education levels, compensation, and retention in the workforce, and to link those elements successfully. Currently, the system is not enticing for these students. Logistical and financial obstacles, from transportation to the cost of books, are constraints. Often students are encouraged to take one-at-a-time courses that do not lead them anywhere, in part because of poor articulation within the higher education systems of most states. Often, "the coursework just isn't very good," in her view. The standards are not there to encourage or to mandate them to get additional education, and when they do, they receive little recognition. Employers are not always supportive of workers who bring best practices back into their programs, and their compensation will not necessarily increase as they acquire more education.

Thus, in her view, a systematic effort is needed to make continuing education accessible, affordable, and of high quality. For her, this is a social justice issue. Some efforts are under way in states, and among national organizations, but they must go further, she added. Six compensation strategies have shown some promise:

- Closed delivery systems, such as the U.S. Department of Defense, that link career ladders, wages, and benefits;
- Requirements for parity in pay and benefits with the prekindergarten sector, as has been tried in a few cases, such as New Jersey's Abbott preschools and public prekindergarten programs in North Carolina;
- Wage subsidies to help child care programs meet minimum salary requirements for different types of work, such as the Washington Career Ladder, and San Francisco's WAGES Plus program;
- Individual salary supplements, now offered by about 15 states, that offer regular, graduated supplements to individuals and are tied to education levels. Examples include Child Care WAGE$® and R.E.W.A.R.D.™[3] WISCONSIN;
- Assistance with health insurance costs—a strategy being used in North Carolina; and
- Comprehensive scholarships such as T.E.A.C.H. Early Childhood®,[4] currently in 22 states and Washington, DC.

Russell also highlighted strategies for improving recognition of these workers. Workforce registries and individual certification are two efforts that states are beginning to adopt. Workforce registries promote profes-

---

[3] Rewarding Education with Wages and Respect for Dedication.
[4] Teacher Education and Compensation Helps Early Childhood.

sional growth and allow states to collect workforce data, while also providing recognition for achievements. Most are voluntary, though Nevada has made registration mandatory by 2012. Individual certification, which is relatively new for ECCE, can also be effective. North Carolina, for example, has a new law that will go into effect in 2012 that requires early educator certification and documents education on a 13-level continuum. Individual licensure, as is required in public schools, combines certification of teacher preparation institutions with a license that grants permission to teach. No state has yet adopted this approach, and licensure occurs most frequently at the center level.

However, Russell explained that most of these strategies are only effective to a certain degree. They are not well funded, are rarely implemented systematically, and are incremental in nature. Bigger solutions are needed, she believes. Her primary recommendation is that teacher compensation must be decoupled from parent fees. Specifically, she advocates that:

- Expectations for professional development and education standards be linked to strategies and funding for increasing compensation;
- States receive or develop funding for an early childhood professional system that is accessible, affordable, and of high quality;
- A public awareness campaign that focuses on the value of investing in effective, well-compensated teachers for young children be mounted;
- Targeted funding streams be developed to support compensation that supplements (1) the costs of teacher education and compensation in exchange for educational progress and retention, and (2) the costs of providing well-educated and fairly compensated teachers in programs that serve low-income families; and
- A special incentive fund be developed for states to reward and support the replication of best practices in early childhood workforce development, compensation, and recognition.

PANEL DISCUSSION ON RECOGNITION OF THE WORKFORCE

A second panel reflected on the issues this presentation raised and offered additional reflections. Ellen Frede, codirector of the National Institute for Early Education Research, focused first on what the early childhood field can do to improve public understanding of its role and its value. Perhaps, she suggested, "we need to let go of some sacred cows." While both public prekindergarten teachers and nurses might be surprised to hear themselves described as well-paid, their wages are higher in comparison with early childhood teachers, and their examples offer some lessons. First, maybe the word "care" should be dropped, Frede suggested, because "care doesn't say we should be paid a lot of money." The distinctions within the early education field—among types of providers, settings, and ages of children—do not serve the field well either, she added. These are important distinctions, but stressing them dilutes the message about how important these experiences are to children and families. Moreover, she added, "I don't know how we get compensation parity if we don't have one system," even if the service is delivered in different ways.

The field also needs to assert itself more firmly, she suggested. "We have to quit accepting the idea that we can use the same amount of money and just spread it over more children or take less money and continue to serve the same number of children." A key to the Abbott Preschool Program's success, she pointed out, was that it defined a set of quality standards from the beginning and refused to deviate from them.

Jana Martella, executive director of the National Association of Early Childhood Specialists in State Departments of Education, agreed that comparisons with the K–12 sector are useful, but noted that that community also has had great frustration over issues of preparation, certification, induction and mentoring, compensation regimes, teacher assessment, and alternate routes to certification.

Shannon Rudisill, director of the Office of Child Care at the Administration for Children and Families, focused on the financial issues. The federal government has made significant recent investments in early education, she observed, but has not found ways to leverage those investments to improve quality. Federal staff frequently consider how many children can be served through a given program at a given cost, but "we have absolutely no model to describe what one more percentage point of quality would look like, or what that would buy," she explained. However, despite these challenges, Rudisill noted the significance of the Patient Protection and Affordable Care Act for the ECCE workforce. "For us to hit 2014, which is only a few years away, and have every single member of the workforce covered by health insurance, will be huge.... I would strongly encourage you to think about the Affordable Care Act as a momentous milestone for our field."

Several workshop participants focused on the demands on this workforce. Kindergarten readiness plays an important role in helping children meet the proficiency goals in the elementary years to which such high stakes are attached, and attention to this set of skills has increased the focus on early education. This, in turn, has highlighted the need to strengthen the early childhood workforce. But "it could take years to get [a workforce] that has the skills and knowledge to be able to get children where they need to be," one noted. The field is still waiting for greater investment in the supports and resources these educators—both prospective and current teachers—need, and for the clearly defined standards that will allow progress to begin, another observed. Many states have begun instituting coaching and mentoring and other supports specifically designed to strengthen teachers' skills, but it may be that, one suggested, "we need scripted curriculums for some members of our workforce—it does provide a scaffold for them." In early education, she added, "we give permission for the program to operate, not to the individual to practice his or her profession." This also probably needs to change, she added, and may require a conversation with the higher education community on a state-by-state basis.

EARLY CHILDHOOD CARE AND EDUCATION AS A PROFESSION

A final panel of discussants provided their views on the future of ECCE as a profession. NAEYC Executive Director Jerlean Daniel said NAEYC is working hard to build the profession, as are other advocates. Their focus is the whole child, she explained, because it is "so easy to focus on particular policies and end up only addressing a very narrow aspect of what children really need to grow and develop." They also work to help people understand that early childhood workers have specialized knowledge, but "it is hard and exhausting work and it never seems to be done." She described a constant "dance between research and practice," but indicated that "really researchers, policy makers, and practitioners must work together."

Linda Smith, executive director of the National Association of Child Care Resource & Referral Agencies, noted that "we don't have a system of health care in this country any more than we have a system of early care and education." In her view, what the early education community can learn from health care is that consumers must be their own advocates as they navigate an array of options that are not really "connected to anything central."

Walter Gilliam, director of the Edward Zigler Center in Child Development and Social Policy at Yale University, echoed this view, suggesting that the difficulty is that even the consumers of the service do not necessarily recognize what constitutes high quality, or what is required to make it possible. One consequence is that "we can't assume that the buyer can actually beware" because the parent—the purchaser—is not in a good position to judge the quality. Compounding this problem is the variability in standards and regulations from state to state. According to Gilliam, the difference between a profession and an occupation is that members of a profession have an identifiable body of knowledge and skills, which most people not only value, but also believe they do not have themselves. However, few people really understand the challenges of working with 3-year-old children, including the knowledge of developmental differences among them, and the skills needed to differentiate pedagogy to address these differences. They assume that because counting and learning preliteracy skills seem simpler than, say, high school mathematics, the teachers of young children have a much easier job than mathematics teachers do. To Gilliam, the lack of understanding and value placed on the work of the ECCE workforce is the crux of the challenge facing the field.

6

Workshop Themes

The workshop planning committee was asked to plan a workshop that would provide an adequate description of the early childhood care and education (ECCE) workforce and outline the parameters that define the population. To better understand the nature of those characteristics, the workshop they planned examined the research on how the workforce affects the development of children, as well as how context shapes the workforce. Presenters examined the challenges and the opportunities that exist within this context to build ECCE as a profession and to support the individuals who provide care and education for young children. This chapter summarizes the main messages from the presentations and discussion on each of these questions, together with key points from the final workshop discussion.

DEFINING AND DESCRIBING THE WORKFORCE

Defining and describing the ECCE workforce is challenging in large part because the purpose and nature of the work, the characteristics of the individuals who do this work, and the settings in which it is done vary a great deal, as discussed in Chapter 2. Care and education are provided in many types of settings, and even those in the field may disagree about its boundaries.

The data available about the workforce vary by type of program and from state to state. This variability and the lack of complete data make it nearly impossible to get a complete picture of the entire ECCE workforce. The presentations and discussions suggested these issues are not only important technical questions pertaining to data collection; they also reflect a lack of precision in the way the field views and organizes itself and conveys to policy makers and the public its value to children and families.

A presenter explored the boundaries within the ECCE workforce, offering definitions of the *occupation* (those paid for direct care and education of young children), the *sector* (those in the occupation plus others employed by the same organizations), and the *enterprise* (those in the sector plus others whose paid work may have a direct influence on caregiving or educational practice). Comments by participants indicated that the field continues to grapple with how to define its borders in a way that is practical but also captures the reality of the work.

Despite the gaps in the available data, presentations identified points that are clear. The workforce is large, accounting for 2.2 million paid workers who make up 30 percent of the total U.S. instructional workforce, including those employed in teaching from early education through higher education (see Chapter 2 and Appendix B). These workers are predominantly female, but they vary by age, race, ethnicity, linguistic and cultural background, family income level, and years of experience, as well as in their expectations and sense of professional identification.

The qualifications these workers bring to the job also vary, and the majority of them have not earned a college degree. These workers vary widely in the degree to which they possess the attitudes, orientations, and skills that have been demonstrated to affect the quality of caregiving and developmental outcomes for children, presentations showed. Compensation is low across the educational spectrum: ECCE workers are poorly compensated in comparison to others with equivalent education.

Several presenters and discussants observed that existing data are not adequate to answer many important policy questions. Federal data systems provide much of the available data, in the form of both large and small one-time studies. Information is also available from registries in some states. The existing federal datasets have advantages. They are well established and permit comparisons of the ECCE workforce with others, and they have produced a valuable body of knowledge. However, decision makers also want more complete information about trends in the characteristics of the workforce as a whole, the influence of market and policy forces on those characteristics, and the relationships between those characteristics and quality of care and outcomes for children.

Workshop discussion highlighted two primary issues that limit the usefulness of existing datasets. First, current guidelines for classifying ECCE workers in federal data systems do not correspond well to the jobs these workers actually do. Second, federal data systems are not designed to capture the detailed information about the workforce that would be useful to policy makers and researchers who want to evaluate the effectiveness of programs, practices, and policies.

In particular, a number of presenters and participants noted, researchers cannot easily use the available data to identify the specific types and levels of training, qualifications, and support that are necessary to achieve the desired levels of quality. These datasets also do not capture differences among types of programs, such as preschool, Head Start, child care, and family child care. More detailed knowledge, participants suggested, could support the design and implementation of workforce development strategies (e.g., compensation, recruitment, retention, pre- and in-service professional development, and ongoing monitoring and support) in a cost-effective manner. Useful models from K–12 education data sources and forward-looking states indicate the need for federal–state partnerships using a combination of sources and types of data collection. Discussion highlighted how improved data collection could bring greater richness and precision to the development of the most cost-effective policies for improving the quality of the workforce and the capacity for monitoring the success of new and existing policies.

THE MARKETPLACE FOR EARLY CHILDHOOD CARE AND EDUCATION WORKERS

Care and education for young children is provided for a fee in an open marketplace. Economic forces have a significant influence on its availability, quality, and cost, as discussed in Chapter 3. There are limits to parents' willingness or capacity to pay more for higher quality of care, economic analysis has shown. At the same time, the supply of people willing to work in early childhood care and education for relatively low wages is elastic, and the field has high rates of job turnover. Thus, despite the tremendous increase in the demand for child care that has occurred as mothers of young children have increased their labor force participation, the wages of ECCE workers have remained relatively flat. Government policies, such as regulations and standards, as well as funding allocations also influence this market. As long as these factors do not change, a presentation made clear, it will be difficult to increase wages enough to attract and retain well-qualified staff, and to encourage existing staff to increase their qualifications.

Research (described in Chapter 3) has demonstrated significant short- and long-term benefits of high-quality care and education for young children, although programs that target disadvantaged children may have larger returns than programs that also serve children who are not disadvantaged. Better datasets and new approaches to calculating the costs and benefits of child care, presentations suggested, hold promise for demonstrating the value of high-quality care and education for all children. Approaches developed for other fields, participants suggested, have helped researchers assign economic value to long-term benefits that are more difficult to measure. Results for a number of early childhood programs indicate that the longest term benefits are generally the greatest—the more data that are accumulated, and the greater the time for benefits to emerge, the greater the quantifiable value of the return on investment. As described in Chapter 3, these analyses are likely to prove particularly useful for policy makers who need to choose among policy alternatives or assess the impact of particular interventions.

EFFECTS ON CHILDREN

Both theory and data indicate that improvements to the quality of the workforce and the workplace will make a difference in outcomes for children, as presenters explained. A variety of research approaches have been used to investigate the relations among caregiver characteristics, the structural features of child care, child care experiences, and children's development (see Chapter 4). Results vary with the age of the children served (e.g., infants, toddlers, preschool-age), and, as in the K–12 sector, it is difficult to isolate specific causal relationships in a complex process. Results from the National Institute of Child Health and Human Development Study of Early Child Care, one study that has explored these connections, showed that higher quality and improved outcomes for very young children were associated with factors such as lower child-to-adult ratios, small group size, and a high-quality physical environment. Caregiver characteristics, such as non-traditional beliefs about child rearing, education and training, experience, conscientiousness, and a positive attitude toward the job, were important predictors of quality for preschoolers. These predictors varied with the ages of the children, and the evidence showed that low child-to-adult ratios are especially important for infants and toddlers.

The benefits to children of high-quality care have been demonstrated empirically (though definitions of quality vary), a presentation made clear, but several discussants noted that the evidence regarding the types of teacher qualifications or experiences likely to yield high-quality care and education is less clear (see Chapter 4). Specifically, inconsistent findings about the value of a bachelor's degree for predicting teacher effectiveness have fueled debate about requirements for teachers. Teacher preparation programs vary widely in quality, and are often reliant on part-time faculty. Other research indicates that training can be quite effective in improving teaching practices. However, discussion suggested that possession of a bachelor's degree, targeted training, or any other single factor alone does not seem to reliably predict high quality. A presenter emphasized that one reason for the equivocal findings is that existing research on the factors that produce desired child outcomes has lacked rigor. Specifically, he stated that more experimental research is needed to understand what teacher and caregiver behaviors and characteristics are causally linked with child outcomes.

Several participants emphasized the need to the search for "silver bullet" solutions. A presenter recommended the evaluation of "packages" of program characteristics associated with a mix of high quality and program effectiveness, which would likely include: well-educated teachers; adequate compensation; strong curriculum and professional development; small classes and reasonable teacher-to-child ratios; good working conditions (paid planning time, substitutes, regular meetings, etc.); strong supervision, monitoring, and review; and both high standards and continuous improvement. Others noted that an environment that allows teachers to apply what they have learned through high-quality preparation and training is also very important.

Researchers have also explored the ways in which racial, ethnic, and language diversity among children and caregivers may influence child outcomes (see Chapter 4). The evidence presented at the workshop suggests that the caregivers' sensitivity and the amount of stimulation provided to children are more important than whether caregivers are similar demographically to the children they care for and educate. However, the research discussed suggested that differences in language background may be more significant, and that children whose home language is not English should have teachers who are bilingual and trained to work with dual-language children.

The conditions in which teachers and caregivers work also have an important influence on outcomes for children, a presentation emphasized. Young children are vulnerable to stress, and continued exposure to situations that cause them to produce high levels of stress hormones can have lasting effects on their development. New research about the specific ways children are affected by stress indicates the profound importance of the quality of the caregiving environment. What is less clear is how to determine the threshold between beneficial care and care that causes stress. Emerging research has pointed to factors—particularly a secure attachment between child and caregiver and the emotional and mental well-being of the caregiver—that are important components of beneficial care. Several presenters and participants suggested that existing quality measures used for licensure and other purposes may not be adequately capturing this critical aspect of care.

Job turnover in ECCE settings is high, a presentation made clear, and highest for the youngest children, who are most vulnerable to lack of stability. Children experience turnover in caregivers as a loss; high turnover also affects the morale of the remaining staff and constrains their ability to work effectively. This circumstance both undermines the quality of care and also reflects aspects of the work environment that are not attractive to highly qualified candidates. Turnover is closely linked with wages. Wage levels in early education and care are very low, in comparison with other fields. Presentations and multiple participants made the point that a supportive workplace that will attract highly motivated and well-qualified workers is one that offers adequate wages and benefits. A supportive workplace is also a learning environment in which workers have the opportunity to discuss and reflect on their work and are empowered to make changes as they learn new practices and skills.

BUILDING THE WORKFORCE

Many presenters and participants emphasized that the early childhood care and education workforce is vitally important to children's well-being and their cognitive, social, and emotional development (see Chapter 5). People who hold these jobs are part of a workforce that has relatively low status and low pay, but the responsibility entrusted to them is extremely serious, as many presenters and participants noted. Making a career in this field more attractive to potential workers, one person observed, will require a large and potentially costly public policy effort to regulate and professionalize the occupation along the lines of public K–12 education. Evidence indicates that such investments can yield substantial improvements in program quality and child development, but presenters and participants suggested that more information about the circumstances in which the benefits exceed the costs is needed.

Moving the ECCE workforce to view itself and function as a profession will be a challenge, many participants noted. Professions are often characterized by entry qualifications, such as a degree and/or a certification, and these requirements are often lacking in ECCE, some observed. As discussed in Chapter 5, other emerging professions, particularly in the health sciences, have shown that the capacity to use data and research to guide changes in standards and practice is essential. Experience in health care suggests that ECCE would benefit if it offered more clearly defined career pathways, based on guidance for students planning their careers, support and mentoring for new teachers, and career ladders that offer financial and other rewards for learning new skills and shouldering new responsibilities. Several presenters pointed to emerging data on promising practices in professional development that can offer empirically based guidance on which features are most important.

Standards exist for training and development and other aspects of quality, but they overlap and are mostly voluntary, presenters and participants noted. Existing systems, several participants and discussants suggested, are also not well integrated across sectors such as child care, Head Start, public prekindergarten, and early intervention programs. Multiple initiatives across these sectors have different funding streams, missions, and standards. If these overlapping segments of the field can be integrated and their efforts coordinated, many participants suggested, the result will be improvements not only in preparation and training for teachers, but also in the quality of the care and education they provide. More than one participant emphasized the importance of ensuring that the needs and roles of the special education community are considered in future coordination efforts.

FILLING THE GAPS

The ECCE field currently does not function as a cohesive system, many presenters and participants observed, and they considered several specific avenues for improvement.

The need for more systematic data collection was a theme noted repeatedly throughout the workshop. Models such as the K–12 public education system and innovative state efforts provide guidance for the development and improvement of early childhood data systems. Participants also identified some goals for both data collection and analytic research.

With regard to data collection systems, various participants noted the value of:

- Reliable estimates of the size and characteristics of the workforce at both the individual occupational level and the organizational or establishment level;
- Data collection that is consistent over time and occurs at frequent enough intervals to capture the effects of changes in economic conditions, major public policy shifts, and other influences;
- The capacity to disaggregate data by state, and, for some information, by local jurisdiction and program type;
- Information about the factors that have been shown to be reliable predictors of quality caregiving, with disaggregation by the ages of children 0 to 5 years; and
- Data that can be used by different actors, including parents, providers, policy makers, and researchers.

Many participants also emphasized that collaborative partnership among federal and state policy makers and private funders is a promising way to implement a coordinated set of data sources, collected on an ongoing basis, to meet these objectives.

Experimental or quasi-experimental studies are also needed, many participants noted, and they highlighted several possible research goals:

- Explore the specific levels of qualifications, working conditions, support, and compensation necessary to recruit and retain a workforce that delivers high-quality care and instruction. That is, provide guidance on the degree of quality improvement that can be expected to produce different types of education and training at varying levels of investment;
- Explore the types and amounts of professional development that are effective in improving the quality of caregiving in different settings and circumstances (e.g., centers versus home care providers);
- Compare the cost-effectiveness of different strategies and techniques for improving the quality of the early childhood workforce;
- Estimate the benefit-to-cost ratios for investments in better qualified and adequately compensated staff, including investments such as professional development activities, rewards for performance, and overall increases in the scale of compensation;
- Measure the impact of market forces, public policy, and societal expectations on the characteristics and performance of the ECCE workforce; and
- Identify relevant similarities or differences in workforce characteristics and needs for children of different age groups (e.g., infants, toddlers, preschoolers), and specific subpopulations (e.g., children with special needs and English-language learners).

FINAL THOUGHTS

Numerous presenters and participants highlighted the importance of the ECCE workforce to the quality of care and education young children receive. They emphasized that while high-quality programs offer great benefits to children and society, care and education that are of poor or even mediocre quality can limit or harm children's development. The varying purposes of and expectations for ECCE, whether focused on enabling parents to work or enhancing child development, have complicated efforts to develop clear occupational definitions, meaningful entry requirements that relate in predictable ways to the quality of care and education, and a cohesive profession, ideas that a number of participants shared during the workshop.

Several participants observed that parents and policy makers alike need a greater understanding of the vital work of the ECCE workforce to help it gain the respect it deserves. As presentations and discussions made clear, this understanding is needed because of the real inherent risks to children in the current system, especially for those in poverty, many of whom participate in settings without teachers and caregivers who are prepared for or supported in their roles. Throughout the workshop, the need for accurate, timely, and meaningful data on the workforce was a theme that repeatedly emerged. Many participants saw better data systems as a critical step toward educating the public about the true nature of the ECCE workforce, targeting ECCE policies efficiently, and knowing whether investments made in the workforce were effective. Many participants recommended that future solutions take into account the context of the workforce, noting that "silver bullet" solutions to challenges do not exist, and that the most successful programs address an array of factors affecting the workforce. In considering how the ECCE workforce might move forward in the future as a profession where the specialized knowledge of early childhood development and pedagogy is developed, recognized, and rewarded, one presenter expressed: "You need the research, you need the data, both [for] the proof, the problem, and to identify the solution. You need individual champions [who are] persistent about their ideas and their goals." Workshop participants were charged to be the leaders of that positive change for the ECCE profession and ultimately for children and families.

References

ACF (Administration for Children and Families). 2006. *Head Start performance measures center. Family and Child Experiences Survey (FACES 2000). Technical report.* HHS-105-96-1912. Washington, DC: U.S. Department of Health and Human Services.

Austin, L. J. E., M. Whitebook, M. Connors, and R. Darrah. 2011. *Staff preparation, reward, and support: Are quality rating and improvement systems addressing all of the key ingredients necessary for change?* Berkeley, CA: Center for the Study of Child Care Employment, University of California, Berkeley.

Badanes, L., M. Mendoza, and S. Watamura. 2011 (unpublished). *Differential susceptibility to stress reactivity at child care for behaviorally inhibited children.* Paper presented at the 2011 Society for Research in Child Development biennial meeting, Montréal, Québec, Canada. University of Denver.

Barbarin, O. A., J. Downer, E. Odom, and D. Head. 2010. Home-school differences in beliefs, support, and control during public pre-kindergarten and their link to children's kindergarten readiness. *Early Childhood Research Quarterly* 25(3):358-372.

Barnett, W. S. 2011. *Preparing highly effective pre-K teachers.* Paper presented at The Early Childhood Care and Education Workforce: A Workshop, Washington, DC, February 28 and March 1.

Barnett, W. S., D. J. Yarosz, J. Thomas, K. Jung, and D. Blanco. 2007. Two-way and monolingual English immersion in preschool education: An experimental comparison. *Early Childhood Research Quarterly* 22(3):277-293.

Bellm, D., and M. Whitebook. 2006. *Roots of decline: How government policy has de-educated teachers of young children.* Berkeley, CA: Center for the Study of Child Care Employment.

Blau, D. M. 1992. The child care labor market. *Journal of Human Resources* 27(1):9-39.

Blau, D. M. 1993. The supply of child care labor. *Journal of Labor Economics* 11(2):324-347.

Blau, D. M. 1997. The production of quality in child care centers. *Journal of Human Resources* 32(2):354-387.

Blau, D. M. 2000. The production of quality in child-care centers: Another look. *Applied Developmental Science* 4(3):136-148.

Blau, D. M. 2001. *The child care problem: An economic analysis.* New York: Russell Sage.

Blau, D. M. 2011. *The economics of early childhood care and education: Implications for the child care workforce.* Paper presented at The Early Childhood Care and Education Workforce: A Workshop, Washington, DC, February 28 and March 1.

Blau, D. M., and A. P. Hagy. 1998. The demand for quality in child care. *Journal of Political Economy* 106(1):104-146.

Blau, D. M., and H. N. Mocan. 2002. The supply of quality in child care centers. *Review of Economics and Statistics* 84(3):483-496.

Brandon, R. N. 2010. *Early care and education workforce logic model developed for the national study of early care and education.* Chicago, IL: National Opinion Research Center, University of Chicago.

Brandon, R. N. 2011. *Counting and characterizing the ECCE workforce.* Paper presented at The Early Childhood Care and Education Workforce: A Workshop, Washington, DC, February 28 and March 1.

Brandon, R. N., and I. Martinez-Beck. 2006. Estimating the size and characteristics of the U.S. early care and education workforce. In *Critical issues in early childhood professional development and training,* edited by M. Zaslow and I. Martinez-Beck. Baltimore, MD: Paul H. Brookes Publishing Co., Inc.

Brandon, R. N., T. J. Stutman, and M. Maroto. 2011. *The economic value of the U.S. early childhood sector.* In Weiss, E. and R. Brandon, 2011, *Economic analysis: The early childhood sector.* Washington, DC: Partnership for America's Economic Success.

Burchinal, M. R., and D. Cryer. 2003. Diversity, child care quality, and developmental outcomes. *Early Childhood Research Quarterly* 18:401-426.

Burchinal, M. R., J. E. Roberts, J. R. Riggins, S. A. Zeisel, E. Neebe, and D. Bryant. 2000. Relating quality of center-based child care to early cognitive and language development longitudinally. *Child Development* 71(2):339-357.

Buysse, V., P. J. Winton, and B. Rous. 2009. Reaching consensus on a definition of professional development for the early childhood field. *Topics in Early Childhood Special Education* 28(4):235-243.

Camilli, G., S. Vargas, S. Ryan, and W. S. Barnett. 2010. Meta-analysis of the effects of early education interventions on cognitive and social development. *Teachers College Record* 112(3):579-620.

Campbell, F. A., and C. T. Ramey. 1995. Cognitive and school outcomes for high risk African American students at middle adolescence: Positive effects of early intervention. *American Educational Research Journal* 32(4):743-772.

Campbell, N. D., J. C. Appelbaum, K. Martinson, and E. Martin. 2000. *Be all that we can be: Lessons from the military for improving our nation's child care system.* Washington, DC: National Women's Law Center.

Clements, D. H., and J. Sarama. 2007. Effects of a preschool mathematics curriculum: Summative research on the building blocks project. *Journal for Research in Mathematics Education* 38(2):136-163.

Dickinson, D. K., and L. Caswell. 2007. Building support for language and early literacy in preschool classrooms through in-service professional development: Effects of the Literacy Environment Enrichment Program (LEEP). *Early Childhood Research Quarterly* 22(2):243-260.

Dower, C., E. H. O'Neil, and H. J. Hough. 2001. *Profiling the professions: A model for evaluating emerging health professions.* San Francisco, CA: Center for the Health Professions, University of California, San Francisco.

Durán, L. K., C. J. Roseth, and P. Hoffman. 2010. An experimental study comparing English-only and transitional bilingual education on Spanish-speaking preschoolers' early literacy development. *Early Childhood Research Quarterly* 25(2):207-217.

Early, D. M., K. L. Maxwell, M. Burchinal, S. Alva, R. H. Bender, D. Bryant, K. Cai, R. M. Clifford, C. Ebanks, J. A. Griffin, G. T. Henry, C. Howes, J. Iriondo-Perez, H.-J. Jeon, A. J. Mashburn, E. Peisner-Feinberg, R. C. Pianta, N. Vandergrift, and N. Zill. 2007. Teachers' education, classroom quality, and young children's academic skills: Results from seven studies of preschool programs. *Child Development* 78(2):558-580.

Farver, J. A. M., C. J. Lonigan, and S. Eppe. 2009. Effective early literacy skill development for young Spanish-speaking English language learners: An experimental study of two methods. *Child Development* 80(3):703-719.

Fowler, S., P. J. Bloom, T. N. Talan, S. Beneke, and R. Kelton. 2008. *Who's caring for the kids? The status of the early childhood workforce in Illinois—2008.* Wheeling, IL: McCormick Tribune Center for Early Childhood Leadership, National-Louis University.

Frede, E. 2011. *Key workforce issues around diversity.* Paper presented at The Early Childhood Care and Education Workforce: A Workshop, Washington, DC, February 28 and March 1.

Frede, E., K. Jung, W. S. Barnett, and A. Figueras. 2009. *The apples blossom: Abbott Preschool Program Longitudinal Effects Study (APPLES), preliminary results through 2nd grade.* New Brunswick, NJ: National Institute for Early Education Research, Rutgers University.

Freedson, M. 2010. Educating preschool teachers to support English language learners. In *Young English language learners: Current research and emerging directions for practice and policy,* edited by E. E. García and E. C. Frede. New York: Teachers College Press. Pp. 165-183.

Fukkink, R. G., and A. Lont. 2007. Does training matter? A meta-analysis and review of caregiver training studies. *Early Childhood Research Quarterly* 22(3):294-311.

García, E., and E. Frede. 2010. *Young English language learners: Current research and emerging directions for practice and policy.* New York: Teacher College Press.

Gebhard, B., S. Ochshorn, and L. Jones. 2010. *Toward a bright future for our youngest children: Building a strong infant-toddler workforce.* Washington, DC: Zero to Three Policy Center.

Gilliam, W. S., and C. M. Marchesseault. 2005. *From capitols to classrooms. Policies to practice: State-funded prekindergarten at the classroom level. Part 1: Who's teaching our youngest students?* New Haven, CT: Yale Child Study Center.

Goe, L., and J. Coggshall. 2007. *The teacher preparation-teacher practices-student outcomes relationship in special education: Missing links and new connections.* Washington, DC: National Comprehensive Center for Teacher Quality.

Goffin, S. G. 2009. *Field-wide leadership: Insights from five fields of practice.* Washington, DC: Goffin Strategy Group.

Gormley, W. T., Jr. 2007. Early childhood care and education: Lessons and puzzles. *Journal of Policy Analysis and Management* 26(3):633-671.

Gunnar, M. R. 2008. Social regulation of stress in early child development. In *Blackwell handbook of early childhood development,* edited by K. McCartney and D. Phillips. Malden, MA: Blackwell Publishing Ltd. Pp. 106-125.

Gunnar, M. R., E. Kryzer, M. J. Van Ryzin, and D. A. Phillips. 2011. The import of the cortisol rise in child care differs as a function of behavioral inhibition. *Developmental Psychology* 47(3):792-803.

Guzman, L., N. D. Forry, M. Zaslow, A. Kinukawa, A. Rivers, A. D. Witte, and R. B. Weber. 2009. *Design phase: National study of child care supply and demand—2010: Literature review and summary.* Prepared for Administration for Children and Families. Washington, DC: U.S. Department of Health and Human Services.

Hamre, B. K., and R. C. Pianta. 2005. Can instructional and emotional support in the first-grade classroom make a difference for children at risk of school failure? *Child Development* 76(5):949-967.

Hanushek, E. A. 2011. The economic value of higher teacher quality. *Economics of Education Review* 30(3):466-479.

Hanushek, E. A., and S. G. Rivkin. 2007. Pay, working conditions, and teacher quality. *The Future of Children* 17(1):69-86.

Heath, S. B. 1989. Oral and literate traditions among black Americans living in poverty. *American Psychologist* 44(2):367-373.

Helburn, S. 1995. *Cost, quality, and child outcomes in child care centers: Technical report.* Denver, CO: Department of Economics, Center for Research in Economic and Social Policy, University of Colorado at Denver.

Herzenberg, S., M. Price, and D. Bradley. 2005. *Losing ground in early childhood education: Declining workforce qualifications in an expanding industry, 1979-2004.* Washington, DC: Economic Policy Institute.

Hock, H., and D. Furtado. 2009. *Female work and fertility in the United States: Effects of low-skilled immigrant labor, working paper 2009-10.* Storrs, CT: University of Connecticut.

Hyson, M., H. B. Tomlinson, and C. A. S. Morris. 2008. Quality improvement in early childhood teacher education: Faculty perspectives and recommendations for the future. *Early Childhood Research & Practice* 11(1). http://ecrp.uiuc.edu/v11n1/hyson.html (accessed August 19, 2011).

Hyson, M., D. Horm, and P. Winton. In press. Higher education for early childhood educators and outcomes for young children: Pathways toward greater effectiveness. In *Handbook of early intervention*, edited by R. Pianta, L. Justice, S. Barnett and S. Sheridan. New York: Guilford Press.

IOM (Institute of Medicine). 1999. *To err is human: Building a safer health system.* Washington, DC: National Academy Press.

Kagan, S. L., K. Kauerz, and K. Tarrant. 2008. *The early care and education teaching workforce at the fulcrum: An agenda for reform.* New York: Teachers College Press.

Karoly, L. A. 2011a. *Toward standardization of benefit-cost analyses of early childhood interventions.* Santa Monica, CA: RAND Corporation.

Karoly, L. A. 2011b. *Using benefit-cost analysis to inform early childhood care and education policy.* Paper presented at The Early Childhood Care and Education Workforce: A Workshop, Washington, DC, February 28 and March 1.

Karoly, L. A., M. R. Kilburn, and J. S. Cannon. 2005. *Early childhood interventions: Proven results, future promise.* Santa Monica, CA: RAND Corporation.

Kelley, P., and G. Camilli. 2007. *The impact of teacher education on outcomes in center-based early childhood education programs: A meta-analysis.* New Brunswick, NJ: National Institute for Early Education Research, Rutgers University.

Kersten, K., E. Frey, and A. Hähnert. 2009. *ELIAS: Early Language and Intercultural Acquisition Studies.* Magdeburg, Germany: EU Education, Audiovisual and Culture Executive Agency.

Kilburn, M. R., and L. A. Karoly. 2008. *The economics of early childhood policy: What the dismal science has to say about investing in children.* Santa Monica, CA: RAND Corporation.

Lambert, R. G., A. Sibley, and R. Lawrence. 2010. Choosing content. In *Preparing teachers for the early childhood classroom: Proven models and key principles*, edited by S. B. Neuman and M. L. Kamil. Baltimore, MD: Paul H. Brookes Publishing Co., Inc.

Lonigan, C., and G. J. Whitehurst. 1998. Relative efficacy of parent and teacher involvement in a shared-reading intervention for preschool children from low-income backgrounds. *Early Childhood Research Quarterly* 13(2):263-290.

Malerba, C. A. 2005 (unpublished). *The determinants of children's and adults' behavioral processes in home and center based child care.* University of Texas at Austin.

Martin, J. N., and N. A. Fox. 2008. Temperament. In *Blackwell handbook of early childhood development*, edited by K. McCartney and D. Phillips. Malden, MA: Blackwell Publishing Ltd. Pp. 126-146.

Maxwell, K. L., C. C. Feild, and R. M. Clifford. 2006. Defining and measuring professional development in early childhood research. In *Critical issues in early childhood professional development*, edited by M. J. Zaslow and I. Martinez-Beck. Baltimore, MD: Paul H. Brookes Publishing Co., Inc. Pp. 21-48.

NAEYC (National Association for the Education of Young Children). 2009. *NAEYC standards for early childhood professional preparation programs*. Washington, DC: NAEYC.

NCATE (National Council for Accreditation of Teacher Education). 2010. *Transforming teacher education through clinical practice: A national strategy to prepare effective teachers*. Washington, DC: NCATE.

NICHD (National Institute for Child Health and Human Development). 1999. Child outcomes when child care center classes meet recommended standards for quality. NICHD Early Child Care Research Network. *American Journal of Public Health* 89(7):1072-1077.

NICHD. 2002. Early child care and children's development prior to school entry: Results from the NICHD Study of Early Child Care. *American Educational Research Journal* 39(1):133-164.

NPDCI (National Professional Development Center on Inclusion). 2008. *What do we mean by professional development in the early childhood field?* Chapel Hill, NC: University of North Carolina at Chapel Hill, FPG Child Development Institute, Author.

NRC (National Research Council). 1990. *Who cares for America's children?: Child care policy for the 1990s*. Washington, DC: National Academy Press.

NRC. 2001. *Eager to learn: Educating our preschoolers*. Washington, DC: National Academy Press.

NRC and IOM (National Research Council and Institute of Medicine). 2000. *From neurons to neighborhoods: The science of early childhood development*. Washington, DC: National Academy Press.

NRC and IOM. 2009. *Strengthening benefit-cost analysis for early childhood interventions: Workshop summary*. Washington, DC: The National Academies Press.

NSCDC (National Scientific Council on the Developing Child). 2005. *Excessive stress disrupts the architecture of the developing brain: Working paper #3*. Cambridge, MA: Center on the Developing Child, Harvard University.

OECD (Organisation for Economic Co-operation and Development). 2006. *Starting strong II: early childhood education and care*. OECD Publishing. doi: 10.1787/9789264035461-en.

OMB (Office of Management and Budget). 2007. *North American Industry Classification System: United States*. Washington, DC: U.S. Government Printing Office.

OMB. 2010. *Standard occupational classification manual, 2010*. Washington, DC: U.S. Government Printing Office.

Peisner-Feinberg, E. S., M. R. Burchinal, R. M. Clifford, M. L. Culkin, C. Howes, S. L. Kagan, and N. Yazejian. 2001. The relation of preschool child-care quality to children's cognitive and social developmental trajectories through second grade. *Child Development* 72(5):1534-1553.

Phillips, D. A., N. A. Fox, and M. R. Gunnar. 2011. Same place, different experiences: Bringing individual differences to research in child care. *Child Development Perspectives* 5(1):44-49.

Pianta, R. C., and M. W. Stuhlman. 2004. Teacher-child relationships and children's success in the first years of school. *School Psychology Review* 33(3):444-458.

Pianta, R. C., K. M. La Paro, and B. K. Hamre. 2005 (unpublished). *Classroom assessment scoring system (class)*. University of Virginia.

Pianta, R. C., A. J. Mashburn, J. T. Downer, B. K. Hamre, and L. Justice. 2008. Effects of web-mediated professional development resources on teacher-child interactions in prekindergarten classrooms. *Early Childhood Research Quarterly* 23(4):431-451.

Pianta, R. C., W. S. Barnett, M. Burchinal, and K. R. Thornburg. 2009. The effects of preschool education. *Psychological Science in the Public Interest* 10(2):49-88.

Powell, D. R., K. E. Diamond, M. R. Burchinal, and M. J. Koehler. 2010. Effects of an early literacy professional development intervention on Head Start teachers and children. *Journal of Educational Psychology* 102(2):299-312.

Richardson, G., and E. Marx. 1989. *A welcome for every child—how France achieves quality in child care: Practical ideas for the United States. The report of the child care study panel of the French-American Foundation.* New York: French-American Foundation.

Rothbart, M. K., M. I. Posner, and J. Kieras. 2006. Temperament, attention, and the development of self-regulation. In *Blackwell handbook of early childhood development*, edited by K. McCartney and D. Phillips. Malden, MA: Blackwell Publishing Ltd. Pp. 338-357.

Ruopp, R., and N. Irwin. 1979. *Children at the center: Summary findings and their implications.* Cambridge, MA: Abt Books.

Schweinhart, L. J., H. V. Barnes, and D. P. Weikart. 1993. *Significant benefits: The High/Scope Perry Preschool Study through age 27. Monograph.* Ypsilanti, MI: High/Scope Educational Research Foundation.

Silvern, S. B. 1988. Continuity/discontinuity between home and early childhood education environments. *The Elementary School Journal* 89(2):147-159.

Sommers, D. 2011. *Federal statistical system.* Paper presented at The Early Childhood Care and Education Workforce: A Workshop, Washington, DC, February 28 and March 1.

Suárez-Orozco, C., and M. M. Suárez-Orozco. 2001. *Children of immigration.* Boston, MA: Harvard University Press.

Wasik, B. A. 2010. What teachers can do to promote preschoolers' vocabulary development: Strategies from an effective language and literacy professional development coaching model. *The Reading Teacher* 63(8):621-633.

Wei, R. C., L. Darling-Hammond, A. Andree, N. Richardson, and S. Orphanos. 2009. *Professional learning in the learning profession: A status report on teacher development in the U.S. and abroad. Technical report.* Oxford, OH: National Staff Development Council.

West, J. 2011. *Learning from NCES and K–12 data systems.* Paper presented at The Early Childhood Care and Education Workforce: A Workshop, Washington, DC, February 28 and March 1.

Whitebook, M. 2003. *Early education quality: Higher teacher qualifications for better learning environments—a review of the literature.* Berkeley, CA: Center for the Study of Child Care Employment, University of California, Berkeley.

Whitebook, M., and S. Ryan. 2011. *Degrees in context: Asking the right questions about preparing skilled and effective teachers of young children.* New Brunswick, NJ: National Institute for Early Education Research, Rutgers University.

Whitebook, M., C. Howes, and D. Phillips. 1990. *Who cares? Child care teachers and the quality of care in America. Final report: National Child Care Staffing Study.* Oakland, CA: Child Care Employee Project.

Whitebook, M., L. Sakai, E. Gerber, and C. Howes. 2001. *Then & now: Changes in child care staffing, 1994-2000. Technical report.* Washington, DC: Center for the Child Care Workforce.

Whitebook, M., D. Phillips, J. Jo, N. Crowell, S. Brooks, and E. Gerber. 2003. *Change and stability among publicly subsidized license-exempt child care providers.* Berkeley, CA: Center for the Study of Child Care Employment, University of California, Berkeley.

Whitebook, M., D. Phillips, D. Bellm, N. Crowell, M. Almaraz, and J. Y. Jo. 2004. *Two years in early care and education: A community portrait of quality and workforce stability, Alameda County, California.* Berkeley, CA: Center for the Study of Child Care Employment, University of California, Berkeley.

Whitebook, M., L. Sakai, F. Kipnis, Y. Lee, D. Bellm, M. Almaraz, and P. Tran. 2006. *California early care and education workforce study: Licensed child care centers and family child care providers statewide highlights, July 2006.* Berkeley, CA & San Francisco, CA: Center for the Study of Child Care Employment, University of California, Berkeley, and California Child Care Resource and Referral Network.

Whitebook, M., L. Sakai, and F. Kipnis. 2010. *Beyond homes and centers: The workforce in three California early childhood infrastructure organizations.* Berkeley, CA: Center for the Study of Child Care Employment, University of California, Berkeley.

Whitebook, M., L. Sakai, F. Kipnis, M. Almarez, E. Suarez, and D. Bellm. 2011. *Learning together: A study of six B.A. completion programs in early care and education—Year 1 report.* Berkeley, CA: Center for the Study of Child Care Employment, University of California, Berkeley.

Winton, P. J., J. A. McCollumn, and C. Catlett. 2008. *Practical approaches to early childhood professional development: Evidence, strategies, and resources.* Washington, DC: Zero to Three Policy Center.

A

Workshop Agenda and Participant List

The Early Childhood Care and Education Workforce: A Workshop

February 28 and March 1, 2011

Georgetown University Conference Center
Thomas and Dorothy Leavey Center
Salons D & E
Georgetown University
Washington, DC

AGENDA

Day 1

8:30 a.m.   Welcoming remarks
Shannon Rudisill, Administration for Children and Families, HHS
Aletha Huston, University of Texas–Austin

Session 1: Defining and Describing the ECCE Workforce

9:00 a.m.   Introduction
A conceptual definition and description of the early childhood care and education workforce
Richard Brandon, RNB Consulting

9:30 a.m.   A framework for ECCE data systems: Current federal data systems and building a federal–state partnership
Richard Brandon, RNB Consulting

9:55 a.m.   Learning from NCES and K–12 data systems
Jerry West, Mathematica Policy Research

Learning from the state-level experience
Harriet Dichter, First Five Years Fund

Discussion

99

10:45 a.m.　　Break

11:00 a.m.　　Economic issues in early care and education

The economics of early childhood care and education
David Blau, The Ohio State University

Short- and long-term costs and benefits of investing in ECCE
Lynn Karoly, RAND Corporation

12:00 p.m.　　Lunch

Session 2: Efficacy: How the ECCE Workforce Affects Children and Families

1:00 p.m.　　Key characteristics of the workforce linked to child and family outcomes

Results from the NICHD Study of Early Childcare
Aletha Huston, University of Texas–Austin

Key workforce issues around cultural diversity
Ellen Frede, National Institute for Early Education Research

2:00 p.m.　　The importance of teacher/caregiver qualifications
Margaret Burchinal, University of North Carolina at Chapel Hill
W. Steven Barnett, National Institute for Early Education Research

3:00 p.m.　　Break

3:15 p.m.　　Research on the nature of working conditions, its impact on teacher well-being, and the relationship with child outcomes
Marcy Whitebook, Center for the Study of Child Care Employment, UC–Berkeley
Deborah Phillips, Georgetown University

4:30 p.m.　　*Joan Lombardi, Administration for Children and Families, HHS*

5:00 p.m.　　Discussion

5:30 p.m.　　Adjourn

Day 2

Session 3: Building the Workforce and the Profession

8:30 a.m.   Opening remarks
A template for evaluating emerging professions
Catherine Dower, Center for the Health Professions,
UC–San Francisco

8:40 a.m.   Discussion regarding the conceptual definition of the
workforce
Richard Brandon, RNB Consulting and Sharon Lynn Kagan,
Columbia University

9:05 a.m.   Framing the issues: Where are we today?
Marcy Whitebook, Center for the Study of Child Care
Employment, UC–Berkeley

9:20 a.m.   Education and training

Overview of key issues and systems in education and
training
Pamela Winton, University of North Carolina at Chapel Hill

Discussant panel:
Tammy Mann, United Negro College Fund
Sharon Ramey, Virginia Tech and Georgetown University
Martha Zaslow, Society for Research in Child Development

10:20 a.m.   Break

10:30 a.m.   "Recognition" of the ECCE workforce: Career ladders,
finance and regulation, overview of the system of
compensation and program funding, and their links with
workforce support and development
Sue Russell, Child Care Services Association

Discussant panel:
Ellen Frede, National Institute for Early Education Research
Jana Martella, National Association of Early Childhood
Specialists in State Departments of Education
Shannon Rudisill, Office of Child Care

11:30 a.m.   Proactive practice and viability of ECCE as a profession: Next steps

Learning from the health care field
*Catherine Dower, Center for the Health Professions,
UC–San Francisco*

Discussant panel:
Jerlean Daniel, National Association for the Education of Young Children
Walter Gilliam, Yale University
Linda Smith, National Association of Child Care Resource and Referral Agencies

12:30 p.m.   Workshop adjourns

PARTICIPANT LIST

Committee Members

Aletha C. Huston, Ph.D. (*Chair*), Priscilla Pond Flawn Regents Professor of Child Development, Human Development and Family Sciences, The University of Texas

David M. Blau, Ph.D., SBS Distinguished Professor of Economics, Department of Economics, The Ohio State University

Richard N. Brandon, Ph.D., Director, Human Services Policy Center, Evans School of Public Affairs, University of Washington

Jeanne Brooks-Gunn, Ph.D., Virginia and Leonard Marx Professor of Child Development, Teachers College and College of Physicians and Surgeons, Columbia University

Virginia Buysse, Ph.D., Senior Scientist, Frank Porter Graham Child Development Center, University of North Carolina at Chapel Hill

Deborah J. Cassidy, Ph.D., Director, Division of Child Development, North Carolina Department of Health and Human Services

Catherine Dower, J.D., Associate Director–Research, Center for the Health Professions, University of California, San Francisco

Yolanda Garcia, M.S., Director, E3 Institute Advancing Excellence in Early Education, WestEd

Sharon Lynn Kagan, Ph.D., Professor of Early Childhood and Family Policy, Teachers College, Columbia University

Robert G. Lynch, Ph.D., Professor of Economics and Interim Chair, Department of Economics, Washington College

Dixie Sommers, M.A., Assistant Commissioner, Occupational Statistics and Employment Projections, Bureau of Labor Statistics, U.S. Department of Labor

Marcy Whitebook, Ph.D., Director and Senior Researcher, Center for the Study of Child Care Employment, University of California, Berkeley

Speakers and Discussants

W. Steven Barnett, Ph.D., Director, National Institute for Early Education Research, Rutgers, The State University of New Jersey

Margaret R. Burchinal, Ph.D., Research Professor and Director, Design and Statistical Computing Unit, University of North Carolina at Chapel Hill

Jerlean E. Daniel, Ph.D., Executive Director, National Association of the Education of Young Children

Harriet Dichter, J.D., National Director, First Five Years Fund

Ellen Frede, Ph.D., Codirector, National Institute for Early Education Research, Rutgers, The State University of New Jersey

Walter Gilliam, Ph.D., Director, The Edward Zigler Center in Child Development and Social Policy, Yale University

Lynn A. Karoly, Ph.D., Senior Economist, RAND Corporation

Joan Lombardi, Ph.D., Office of the Assistant Secretary, Administration for Children and Families, HHS

Tammy Mann, Ph.D., Executive Director, Frederick D. Patterson Research Institute, United Negro College Fund

Jana Martella, M.S., Executive Director, National Association of Early Childhood Specialists in State Departments of Education and National Association for Regulatory Administration

Deborah A. Phillips, Ph.D., Professor, Department of Psychology, Georgetown University

Sharon Ramey, Ph.D., Director, Susan H. Mayer Professor for Child and Family Studies, School of Nursing, Georgetown University

Shannon Rudisill, M.S.W., Associate Director, Child Care Bureau, Office of Child Care, Administration for Children and Families, HHS

Susan D. Russell, President, Child Care Services Association

Linda K. Smith, Executive Director, National Association of Child Care Resource & Referral Agencies

Jerry West, Ph.D., Senior Fellow, Mathematica Policy Research

Pamela J. Winton, Ph.D., Senior Scientist, Director of Outreach, FPG Child Development Institute, University of North Carolina at Chapel Hill

Martha Zaslow, Ph.D., Director, Office for Policy and Communications, Society for Research in Child Development

Guests

Patrick Aaby, Policy Advisor to the Executive Director, Committee for Children

Jane Banister, Director, Hoya Kids Learning Center

Stacie Beland, Professional Advancement Project Director, Edward Street Child Services

Paula Bendl Smith, Child Care Specialist, Office of Child Care, Administration for Children and Families, HHS

Soumya Bhat, Senior Program Associate, The Finance Project

Natacha Blain, Associate Director, Grantmakers for Children, Youth & Families

Carole Brown, Research Associate Professor, Catholic University

Sherry Burke, Director of Programs and Research, Committee for Children

Kelly Burnes, Project Associate, NYC Early Childhood Professional Development Institute, City University of New York

Beth Caron, Education Program Specialist, U.S. Department of Education

Rita Catalano, Executive Director, Fred Rogers Center at Saint Vincent College

Jamie Colvard, State Policy Analyst, Zero to Three

Theresa Cosca, Economist, Bureau of Labor Statistics, U.S. Department of Labor

Elise Crane, Senior Program & Policy Analyst, San Francisco Human Services Agency

Bethlehem Dammlash, Grantmakers for Children, Youth & Families

Karen Davis Platt, Quality Improvement Manager, National Association of Child Care Resource & Referral Agencies

Kathy Edler, Head Start Fellow, Office of Child Care, Administration for Children and Families, HHS

Sarah Friedman, Research Director, CNA Corporation

Sara Gable, Associate Professor, University of Missouri

Dorothy Gibson, Consultant, American Federation of Teachers

Linda Gillespie, TA Specialist, Zero to Three

Stacie Goffin, Principal, Goffin Strategy Group

Tamara Halle, Senior Research Scientist, Child Trends

Karen Heying, Project Director, National Infant & Toddler Child Care Initiative, Zero to Three

Steven Hicks, Office of the Secretary, U.S. Department of Education

Mimi Howard, Head Start Fellow, Office of Head Start, Administration for Children and Families, HHS
Inette Hunter, Implementation Associate, Teaching Strategies, Inc.
Joanne Hurt, Executive Director, Wonders Child Care
Alicia Jaramillo-Underwood, Board on the Health of Select Populations, Institute of Medicine
Shelby Kain, Analyst, U.S. Government Accountability Office
Eric Karolak, Executive Director, Early Care and Education Consortium
Eugenia Kemble, Executive Director, Albert Shanker Institute
Fran Kipnis, Research Specialist, Center for the Study of Child Care Employment, University of California, Berkeley
Rose Kor, Wyoming Children's Action Alliance
Sarah Lacey, Director of Provider Support Services, Indiana Association for Child Care Resource and Referral
Beth Ann Lang, Project Coordinator, T.E.A.C.H. Early Childhood Missouri Scholarship
Sarah LeMoine, Director, State Workforce Systems Policy, National Association for the Education of Young Children
Morgan Ludlow, Economist, U.S. Bureau of Labor Statistics
Elizabeth Manlove, Associate Professor, Lock Haven University
Laura Martinez, Senior Program Associate, The Finance Project
Ivelisse Martinez-Beck, Senior Social Science Research Analyst, Office of Planning, Research & Evaluation, Administration for Children and Families, HHS
Janet Mascia, Assistant Director, U.S. Government Accountability Office
Caitlin McLaughlin, National Association of Child Care Resource & Referral Agencies
Kimberly Means, Head Start Fellow, Office of Head Start, Administration for Children and Families, HHS
Mary Mueggenborg, Social Science Research Analyst, Office of Planning, Research & Evaluation, Administration for Children and Families, HHS
Carol Nolan, National Head Start Fellow, Office of Head Start, Administration for Children and Families, HHS
Sue Offutt, Executive Director, McCormick Center for Early Childhood Leadership
Ngozi Onunaku, Senior Policy Analyst, Administration for Children and Families, HHS
Cassandra Piper, Quality Improvement Manager, National Association of Child Care Resource & Referral Agencies
Michele Plutro, Office of Head Start, Administration for Children and Families, HHS
Esther Quintero, Albert Shanker Institute

Darlene Ragozzine, Executive Director, Connecticut Charts-A-Course
Craig Ramey, Distinguished Scientist and Professor, Virginia Tech
    Carilion Research Institute
Carla Rojas, Analyst, U.S. Government Accountability Office
Pattie Ryan, Deputy Director, Indiana Association for Child Care
    Resource and Referral
Jessica Sabol, Associate, American Federation of Teachers
Mary Beth Salomone Testa, Policy Director, Early Care and Education
    Consortium
Roberta Schomburg, Associate Dean, School of Education, Carlow
    University
Oman Shamind, National Head Start Fellow
Julie Shuell, Director, National Child Care Information and Technical
    Assistance Center
Jill Soto, The National Registry Alliance
Lauren Supplee, Senior Social Science Research Analyst, Administration
    for Children and Families, HHS
Maria Taylor, CEO, ChildCare Education Institute
Suzanne Thouvenelle, Subject Matter Specialist, Head Start Knowledge
    Information Management
Melodie Vega, Project Manager, Hawaii Careers with Young Children
Jere Wallden, The National Registry Alliance
Mary Bruce Webb, Director, Division of Child and Family
    Development, Office of Planning, Research & Evaluation,
    Administration for Children and Families, HHS
Jennifer Weber, Manager of Policy, Nemours
Emily Wengrovius, Policy Specialist, National Conference of State
    Legislatures
T'Pring R. Westbrook, Office of Planning, Research & Evaluation,
    Administration for Children and Families, HHS
Greg Yorker, Director, T.E.A.C.H. Early Childhood Ohio, Ohio Child
    Care Resource & Referral Association
Marcy Young, Pew Center on the States

Project Staff

Rosemary Chalk, Director, Board on Children, Youth, and Families
Holly Rhodes, Study Director, Board on Children, Youth, and Families
Alexandra Beatty, Rapporteur
Reine Homawoo, Senior Program Assistant, Board on Children, Youth,
    and Families
Wendy Keenan, Program Associate, Board on Children, Youth, and
    Families

Appendix B

Commissioned Papers

SUMMARY OF BACKGROUND DATA ON THE ECCE
WORKFORCE
Michelle L. Maroto and Richard N. Brandon

Prepared for the IOM Committee on the ECCE Workforce

INTRODUCTION AND PURPOSE

The National Research Council and Institute of Medicine (IOM) convened a Committee on the Early Childhood Care and Education Workforce, which is charged with holding a workshop to provide a clear definition of who is included in that workforce and to explore major issues regarding how to support the workforce and improve the quality of services it provides. A first step in that effort is to summarize the number and characteristics of the early childhood care and education (ECCE) workforce. This paper summarizes the currently available information about the number and characteristics of the ECCE workforce in the United States drawing mostly on published studies, tabulations from federal databases, and survey data compiled from multiple studies. Some previously unpublished data from several federal data sources provided by the U.S. Bureau of Labor Statistics have been included.

The first challenge in this task comes from the lack of a uniformly accepted definition of the ECCE workforce, with many studies including workers who are not within the relevant standard federal occupational definitions and excluding others who are paid for similar work. This paper takes the approach first developed by Brandon and Whitebook for estimating the number of ECCE workers,[1] which treats any individual who is paid for the care and education of children age birth through five and not in kindergarten as a member of the ECCE workforce. The definition of ECCE workforce used is derived from focusing on the function of being paid to provide care or instruction for young children, regardless of the setting or program in which it occurs. This definition is consistent with the federal concept of what constitutes an occupation, which is independent of the location in which the occupation is carried out.

It is common to divide ECCE into three broad categories reflecting the type of setting in which care and instruction occur: center-based (including community-based centers, preschools, and Head Start programs); formal home-based or Family Child Care (FCC), in which "formal" refers to being available in the open market and often licensed or registered; and informal home-based or Family, Friend, and Neighbor (FFN) care, where there is a relationship between the child and caregiver and access is not broadly available in the community. However, there are not clear demarcations among these types of settings. Family Child Care homes are often expanded to include many children and several staff, and are not distinguishable from small centers; some FFN caregivers function as small businesses not clearly separable from FCC.

In all three settings, some care or instruction is provided by unpaid individuals, who are not normally considered part of a workforce. An appropriate estimate of the size of the workforce therefore requires the ability to distinguish between paid and unpaid care and instruction. Because of the overlap and presence of unpaid caregivers, these three categories therefore serve as useful descriptors, but do not clearly define who is or is not included in the ECCE workforce.

We were able to identify 50 relevant studies providing information regarding the size and characteristics of the ECCE workforce. This summary presents broad findings regarding the numbers and characteristics of the ECCE workforce as suggested by these 50 studies, plus additional characteristics derived from several federal data sources provided by Dixie Sommers and Theresa Cosca at the U.S. Bureau of Labor Statistics (BLS). A description of these studies and their citations may be found at the end of this summary report. Detailed matrices summarizing the find-

---

[1] A. Burton, R. N. Brandon, E. Maher, M. Whitebook, M. Young, D. Bellm, and C. Wayne, *Estimating the Size and Components of the U.S. Child Care Workforce and Caregiving Population* (Center for the Child Care Workforce [CCW] and Human Services Policy Center [HSPC], May 2002).

ings from the national and state studies will be made available on the IOM project website.

Twenty-five of these studies used national samples, and the rest came from different state-level studies. Because comprehensive surveys of the ECCE workforce that use nationally representative samples are rare, we combine multiple studies in our summary to present a broad picture of workers. This picture is partial, and we acknowledge a need for more recent representative data about the ECCE workforce.

In this summary, we relied on recent studies that provided the best descriptive information about workers. Generally, state-level studies provided the most detailed information, but we refrain from including them in this summary paper because they are not necessarily representative of the U.S. population. Two reviews of state workforce studies found wide variation in the robustness of methodology employed[2] and in the reported levels of such essential characteristics as educational attainment.[3]

Much of this summary is based on new, unpublished tabulations of federal workforce data reflecting federal occupation and industry codes used by the BLS and the Census Bureau. We requested these data because the most recent nationally representative surveys of the ECCE workforce were conducted between 10 to 20 years ago.

We also include characteristics of subsets of the ECCE workforce from more recent, but limited, studies when items of interest are not available from nationally representative sources. Most of the federal databases and studies on the ECCE workforce were lacking in different ways, which complicates the summary. What we present is therefore somewhat of a "pastiche," combining the best available data from numerous sources to address key questions. We have excluded any data that we consider unreliable or unrepresentative.

Michelle Maroto of the University of Washington identified 50 relevant studies, which we have divided into seven categories reflecting their relative strength for describing the characteristics of the ECCE workforce on a national scale. In order to address study limitations, but still present characteristics of the ECCE workforce, we ranked each study based upon the representativeness of its sample and the types of workers and settings it covered. The sampling structure of studies ranged from nationally

---

[2] G. Stahr-Breunig, R. N. Brandon, and E. J. Maher, "Counting the Child Care Workforce: A Catalog of State Data Sources to Quantify and Describe Child Caregivers in the Fifty States and the District of Columbia," report to the Child Care Bureau, Administration for Children and Families, U.S. Department of Health and Human Services, February 2004.

[3] R. N. Brandon and I. Martinez-Beck, "Estimating the Size and Characteristics of the U.S. Early Care and Education Workforce," in *Critical Issues in Early Childhood Professional Development and Training*, ed. M. Zaslow and I. Martinez-Beck (Brooks Publishing Company, 2005).

representative samples to multistate samples to state-level representative samples. The different settings of interest include center- and home-based care. In addition, studies used different language to refer to child care workers. Some studies divided child care workers into teachers, assistant teachers, and aids. Others only had divisions for center workers and FCC workers. Still others took a limited focus and only surveyed preschool teachers.

The studies summarized at the end of this report are categorized below; the number of studies in each category is shown in parenthesis:

I.   *Nationally representative; cover all children age B–5 (birth–age 5) and distinguish B–5 from school age; include most settings (2)*

    1. Profile of Child Care Settings (PCCS), 1990
    2. National Households Education Survey (NHES); Human Services Policy Center (HSPC)/Center for the Child Care Workforce (CCW) Child Care Workforce Estimates Study, 2005

II.   *Nationally representative; include most settings; cover all B–5 but do not distinguish from school-age (7)*

    1. Current Population Survey (CPS), 2004
    2. CPS; Occupation, 2010
    3. CPS; Industry, 2010
    4. American Community Survey (ACS); Occupation, 2009
    5. ACS; Industry, 2009
    6. Quarterly Census of Employment and Wages (QCEW), 2009
    7. American Time Use Survey (ATUS); HSPC Estimating the Economic Value of Early Care and Education, 2005–2007

III.   *Nationally representative; cover a portion of B–5 workforce or settings; e.g., prekindergarten, Head Start (7)*

    1. Head Start Impact Study (HSIS), 2002–2006
    2. Head Start: The Family and Child Experiences Survey (FACES), 2006–2007
    3. Head Start: FACES, 2001
    4. Head Start: FACES, 2000
    5. Head Start: FACES, 1997
    6. National Prekindergarten Study (NPS), 2003–2004
    7. National Center for Early Development and Learning Survey (NCEDL-S), 1997

IV. *Multistate; cover all of B–5 workforce by child age and setting (4)*

    1. National Child Care Staffing Study (NCCSS), 1988
    2. Cost, Quality and Child Outcomes in Child Care Centers (CQCO), 1993
    3. National Day Care Study (NDCS), 1976–1977
    4. National Day Care Home Study (NDCHS), 1980

V. *Multistate; cover portion of B–5 workforce and settings; e.g., prekindergarten (5)*

    1. National Institute of Child Health and Human Development (NICHD) Study of Early Child Care and Youth Development (SECCYD), 15 Months
    2. NICHD SECCYD, 24 Months
    3. NICHD SECCYD, 36 Months
    4. Multi-State Study of Pre-Kindergarten (MSSPK), 2001
    5. Statewide Early Education Programs Survey (SWEEP), 2001–2003

VI. *Single state; cover all B–5 workforce (21)*

VII. *Single state; cover portion of B–5 workforce and settings; e.g., prekindergarten (4)*

The first ranking tier includes studies that are: (1) nationally representative, (2) cover all child care workers for children birth through age 5, and (3) include most study settings. Within Tier I, the 1990 PCCS was the only study that was drawn from a nationally representative sample, covered child care workers for children birth through 5 years of age, and distinguished them from caregivers of school-aged children. It did not include the large FFN component of the workforce. However, this study was conducted in 1990, which makes it 20 years old and decreases its relevance for workers today. The HSPC analysis conducted in 2011 also meets these specifications, and includes the FFN component, but it only provides estimates of the size of the workforce and does not describe characteristics. Thus, we use the HSPC study for estimates of the size of the ECCE workforce, but rely on other studies to describe the characteristics of the workforce.

Most of the data presented in this report come from studies in the second category. This tier includes studies that are nationally representative and cover all child care workers for children birth through age 5, but do not distinguish these workers from those responsible for school-aged children. Characteristics of child care workers provided by these studies come from Census occupational and industry classifications. We draw on previously unpublished tabulated data from the 2009 and 2010 CPS and the 2009 and 2010 ACS, and data from the HSPC demand-based estimate (Brandon et al., 2011), which used the 2005–2007 ATUS; this allowed identification of Family, Friend, or Neighbor caregivers. The application of federal occupation and industry codes in the surveys on which these studies were based allows us to report some descriptive information that is nationally representative. However, these data also include caregivers for school-aged children. We have only included such data where we do not think there is a likely systematic difference between the characteristics of caregivers of young children and those of school age.

The third tier consists of nationally representative studies that cover only a portion of the ECCE workforce. Thus, they yield information about some groups of child care workers and early education teachers, but not all of them. Some of the data come from the HSIS, which was conducted from 2002–2006 and the Head Start: FACES surveys from 1997 through 2001. Teachers and assistant teachers in these studies were all recruited from Head Start classrooms. This tier also includes the NPS and the NCEDL-S. Both of these studies only surveyed prekindergarten teachers and are thus restricted to children between ages 3 and 5. It should be noted that due to federal and state prekindergarten program standards, the educational level of the prekindergarten workforce reflected in these studies is higher than for the ECCE workforce in general.

The fourth tier consists of multistate studies that cover all of the B–5 child care workforce. Multistate studies often attempted to approximate a nationally representative sample by surveying workers in a diverse subset of states, but none has a sufficient number of states to effectively represent all regions of the United States. The 1988 NCCSS surveyed center workers in five cities (Atlanta, Boston, Detroit, Phoenix, and Seattle). The 1993 CQCO surveyed staff in 400 programs across four states (California, Colorado, Connecticut, and North Carolina). The 1976–1977 NDCS was constructed from state licensing lists and thus systematically underrepresents unlicensed settings and providers in states that only require licensing of a small fraction of providers. The 1980 NDCHS consists of both regulated and unregulated family day care homes in three urban areas (Los Angeles, Philadelphia, and San Antonio). Most of these studies are older; therefore, we do not include much information from them in this report.

The fifth tier consists of multistate studies that cover only a portion of the ECCE workforce. The NICHD SECCYD at 15, 24, and 36 months surveyed caregivers for children in the NICHD study when the children were 15, 24, and 36 months old and thus excluded workers caring only for children above that age. The 2001 MSSPK and the 2001–2003 SWEEP were both conducted by the National Center for Early Development and Learning (NCEDL). The MSSPK is based on a stratified random sample of teachers in state-funded prekindergarten classrooms from six states (California, Georgia, Illinois, Kentucky, New York, and Ohio). The SWEEP was based on state-funded prekindergarten classrooms from five states (Massachusetts, New Jersey, Texas, Washington, and Wisconsin).

The sixth and seventh tiers contain 25 single-state studies from 15 states at different time periods. We do not discuss these data in this summary, but these studies are included in the detailed data matrices. The detailed matrices provide the findings from these studies in much richer detail and discuss the nature of the studies, indicating their strengths and weaknesses for this purpose (which may not have been the primary purpose for which the studies were conducted). The print matrices provide an overview of this information, but the digital file includes estimates for each of the individual studies.

COUNTING THE ECCE WORKFORCE FOR CHILDREN AGE B–5, BY SETTING

The only study that encompassed and distinguished the workforce responsible for children B–5 and included all settings (center-based, formal home-based, and informal home-based) was the HSPC demand-based estimate (Brandon et al., 2011). This study updated and refined earlier work led by Brandon and Whitebook (CCW and HSPC, 2002). This approach is labeled demand-based because the essential data are derived from one of several large scale, nationally representative surveys that ask parents how many hours in a typical week each of their children spends in each type of non-parental care setting, including both formal and FFN care; and whether the care and instruction is paid or unpaid. The National Household Education Survey, Early Childhood Supplement (2005) was deemed most appropriate because it contains the most comprehensive and well-differentiated set of categories for type of care. It also asks parents the child:adult ratio for the setting where their child is in care. The demand-based estimate combines hours per child in care, child:adult ratios and average hours worked by ECE staff (from BLS Current Employment Statistics) to derive the full-time equivalent (FTE) number of adults caring for young children. Because the estimates are derived from samples of individual children with such known characteristics as age, it is possible to divide the workforce by such variables as the age of child and setting. Various other adjustments are made to convert FTEs to individuals and estimate the number of directors and other staff positions associated with that number of caregivers.

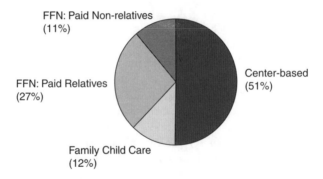

FFN: Paid Non-relatives (11%)

FFN: Paid Relatives (27%)

Center-based (51%)

Family Child Care (12%)

FIGURE B-1 Demand-based estimates of the ECCE workforce.

TABLE B-1 Formal ECCE Workforce by Role/Responsibility

Total Persons in Typical Week	Center-Based Staff				FCC Staff	
	Center Staff: Total	Directors/ Administrators	Teachers	Assistant Teachers and Aides	FCC Providers	FCC Assistants
1,333,000	1,083,000	83,000	564,000	435,000	151,000	99,000

NOTE: ECCE: Early Childhood Care Education; FCC: Family Child Care.
SOURCE: HSPC demand-based estimates. Brandon et al., 2011.

These demand-based estimates are illustrated in Figure B-1. It should be noted that in addition to the 2.2 million paid ECCE workers shown here, the same estimates indicate an additional 3.2 unpaid workers, for a total caregiving population of 5.5 million.

Table B-1 provides a differentiation of the formal components of the ECCE workforce by role or responsibility. The FFN component is not shown because such a differentiation is not relevant.

An advantage of the demand-based approach is that it differentiates by the age of children served as well as by type of setting, as shown in Table B-2. It is useful to differentiate by age of children since different skills and orientations may be required to best meet children's needs.

Differentiation by Occupation and Industry: BLS and Census Bureau Employment Data

The demand-based workforce estimates in the previous section have the advantages of covering all components of the ECCE workforce and

TABLE B-2 Estimated Number of Paid ECCE Workers in the United States in a Typical Week by Setting and Age of Child

	Total Paid	Center Care	FCC Providers	Paid Relatives	Paid Non-Relatives
Infants (0–18 mos.)	490,000	223,000	78,000	111,000	78,000
Toddlers (19–36 mos.)	654,000	309,000	92,000	166,000	87,000
Early Head Start	13,000	13,000			
Private pre-schoolers (3–5 yrs)	826,000	371,000	80,000	312,000	63,000
Public pre-schoolers (3–5 yrs)	79,000	79,000			
Head Start	94,000	94,000			
All 0–5 year olds	2,157,000	1,088,000	250,000	589,000	229,000

NOTE: FCC: Family Child Care.
SOURCE: HSPC demand-based estimates. Brandon et al., 2011.

of being restricted to caring for or instructing children age B–5. However, these estimates have many limitations. They can only be conducted at broad intervals when a demand survey is available. They also entail great uncertainty because they must link many different estimates from different data sources. Because they do not directly interview employees or employer, they lack many essential features included in standard federal workforce data such as the sector or industry in which they are employed, the number of hours worked, wages earned, separation or turnover rate. They also lack the educational and demographic characteristics of members of different occupations collected by the Census Bureau using the same federal occupational classification. In this section, and in Tables B-3A and B-3B below, we draw on relevant federal workforce data from the BLS to complete this initial portrait. In the next major section of the paper, we summarize studies using Census data to provide additional characteristics.

There are many challenges to using standard federal data from the BLS and the Census Bureau to describe the ECCE workforce, as discussed in *Federal Data Sources for Understanding the Early Childhood Care and Education Workforce: A Background Paper*, a second commissioned work included in this report. The primary challenge is that for the largest share of the ECCE workforce, the federal occupational categorization does not differentiate between those employed to provide care and instruction to young children (B–5) and those responsible for school-aged children. However, there are several relevant pieces of data for which there is no particular reason to assume a different distribution of characteristics related to the age of children in care. It is therefore useful to examine those data, keeping in mind this caveat.

Relating ECCE Occupations and Industries

A particular advantage of the federal data system is that it cross-tabulates occupations with the industries or economic sectors in which they are employed. We can thus see that ECCE does not function as an isolated bubble in the U.S. economy, but is highly interwoven with other sectors. Tables B-3A and B-3B are based on BLS employment statistics, as opposed to the demand-based estimates shown in Tables B-1 and B-2. We also compare the size of the ECCE workforce as indicated by each of these sources.

Comparing BLS Employment Estimates to Demand-Based Estimates

As seen in Table B-3A, BLS identified 1.8 million jobs, of which 1.3 million are classified as child care workers and 0.5 million as preschool teachers.

The demand-based estimate exclusive of FFN caregivers was about 1.4 million. Because the BLS estimate of 1.8 million includes caregivers for school-aged children, it would be expected to be larger than the demand-based estimate for children under age 6. If, for example, one-third of child care workers identified by the BLS are working with school-aged children, that would reduce the 1.8 million to 1.3 million. The two estimates are therefore roughly similar for the components of the ECCE workforce that they share.

However, because the BLS estimate probably does not include most of the 0.8 million paid FFN workers in the demand-based estimate, it is reasonable that the 1.8 million is lower than the 2.2 million total in the demand-based estimate. If the 0.8 million demand-based estimate of paid FFN workers is added to the 1.3 million derived from assuming one-third of child care workers care only for school-aged children, the adjusted total would be 2.1 million, roughly comparable to the demand-based estimate of 2.2 million.

Industries Employing ECCE Workers

Of the 1.8 million employees reported by the BLS, 75 percent or 1.3 million are wage and salary employees, and the remaining 431,000 are self-employed, presumably as FCC proprietors. About 247,000 of the wage and salary employees are employed in private households. This estimate could include nannies and some paid FFN caregivers. Subtracting this number from the total wage and salary employees leaves a subtotal of 631,000 individuals who are employed out of the home, plus an additional 390,000 preschool teachers.

The balance between wage and salary and self-employment varies substantially between those classified as child care workers and those as preschool teachers. Almost a third of the child care workers are self-employed, compared to less than 2 percent of preschool teachers.

The industries employing child care workers and preschool teachers are quite different. Of interest is that only about 66,000 or 15 percent of preschool teachers work in public or private schools. More than two-thirds—69 percent—are in social assistance establishments. Presumably Head Start teachers who are employed by community-based contractors are considered social assistance employees.

Within the 631,000 child care workers whose employment is not home-based, the greatest number—253,000—work in child care services, what are commonly thought of as child care centers. But these workers comprise less than a third of such employees.

Child care workers are distributed across a wider range of economic sectors than preschool teachers. About 21 percent are in social assistance; 4 percent in health care, mostly residential facilities; 19 percent are in child day care services, such as community-based centers; 3 percent are in fitness and recreation centers, and 6 percent work for "religious, grantmaking, civic, professional, and similar organizations," which are presumably centers operated by such entities. Less than 1 percent are in transportation (including school-bus drivers) and hotel or motel accommodations.

Almost 50,000 are employed in "residential care facilities," of which the largest number—17,000—are in mental health, mental retardation, and substance abuse facilities. However, we cannot determine whether these workers are responsible for young children of parents residing in such facilities, for adolescent residents, or a combination of the two. This is one of the challenges of not differentiating child care workers by the age group of children served. Because such residential facilities are categorized within the health sector, they would not normally be identified as related to ECCE if the occupations were not specified within the sector.

This brief summary illustrates the value of the BLS system of relating occupations to industries. It allows policy makers to consider both how many employees there are and where they are employed. If large-scale

TABLE B-3A Employment by Occupation and Industry, 2008

| | Child Care Workers | |
| | 2008 | |
Industry	Employment (thousands)	Percentage of Occupation
Total employment, all workers	1,301.9	100.00
Self-employed and unpaid family workers, all jobs	424.0	32.57
Total wage and salary employment	877.8	67.43
Transportation and warehousing (school and employee bus transportation)	11.6	0.89
Educational services, public and private	147.7	11.34
Health care and social assistance	334.2	25.67
Health care	57.3	4.40
Residential care facilities (mental retardation, mental health, substance abuse, other)	49.5	3.80
Social assistance	276.9	21.27
Individual, family, community, and vocational rehabilitation services	23.2	1.79
Child day care services	253.7	19.48
Arts, entertainment, and recreation (including fitness and recreation centers)	34.9	2.68
Amusement, gambling, and recreation industries	34.8	2.68
Accommodation (hotels, motels) and food services	1.0	0.08
Other services (except government and private households)	77.9	5.99
Religious, grantmaking, civic, professional, and similar organizations	77.5	5.96
Government	17.6	1.35
Private households; all jobs	246.5	18.93

NOTE: CC: Child Care.
SOURCE: Bureau of Labor Statistics, Employment Projections, 2009.

quality improvement efforts are being planned, then knowing which establishments employ how many workers is essential.

Employment Projections

Obviously, if policy makers are looking to provide supports and incentives for professional development and quality improvement, locating the

Preschool Teachers		CC Workers + Pre-K	
2008		2008	
Employment (thousands)	Percentage of Occupation	Employment (thousands)	Percentage of Occupation
457.2	100.00	1,759.1	100.00
7.0	1.53	431.0	24.50
450.2	98.47	1,328.0	75.49
		11.6	0.66
66.3	14.51	214.0	12.17
317.3	69.40	651.5	37.04
2.8	0.62	60.1	3.42
0.5	0.10	50.0	2.84
314.5	68.78	591.4	33.62
17.4	3.81	40.6	2.31
297.1	64.97	550.8	31.31
0.7	0.16	35.6	2.02
0.6	0.13	35.4	2.01
		1.0	0.06
58.5	12.80	136.4	7.75
58.5	12.80	136.0	7.73
5.5	1.19	23.1	1.31
0.3	0.07	246.8	14.03

places that employ workers is essential to arranging supports. Planning for both pre-service and in-service professional development, as well as for recruitment activities, is aided by projecting future job growth in different occupations and industries. BLS creates projections regularly for all occupations and industries, considering a variety of economic trends and factors. Table B-3B summarizes the BLS employment projections for

TABLE B-3B Projected Employment by Occupation and Industry, 2018

Industry	Child Care Workers	
	2018	
	Employment (thousands)	Percentage Change
Total employment, all workers	1,443.9	10.91
Self-employed and unpaid family workers, all jobs	445.0	4.93
Total wage and salary employment	999.0	13.80
Transportation and warehousing (school and employee bus transportation)	13.9	19.83
Educational services, public and private	180.3	22.12
Health care and social assistance	375.2	12.27
Health care	63.1	10.24
Residential care facilities (mental retardation, mental health, substance abuse, other)	54.1	9.40
Social assistance	312.1	12.69
Individual, family, community, and vocational rehabilitation services	28.0	20.44
Child day care services	284.1	11.98
Arts, entertainment, and recreation (including fitness and recreation centers)	39.8	14.23
Amusement, gambling, and recreation industries	39.8	14.22
Accommodation (hotels, motels) and food services	1.1	7.75
Other services (except government and private households)	88.5	13.58
Religious, grantmaking, civic, professional, and similar organizations	88.0	13.54
Government	19.0	8.12
Private households; all jobs	273.3	10.88

NOTE: CC: Child Care
SOURCE: Bureau of Labor Statistics, Employment Projections, 2009.

ECCE workers, which incorporate both child care workers (which include school-aged care) and preschool teachers.

We examine ECCE employment by industry or sector because BLS projects employment growth at different rates for sectors reflecting

Preschool Teachers 2018		CC Workers + Pre-K 2018	
Employment (thousands)	Percentage Change	Employment (thousands)	Percentage Change
543.9	18.95	1,987.8	13.00
7.4	5.50	452.4	4.97
536.5	19.16	1,535.5	15.63
		13.9	19.83
72.7	9.53	253.0	18.22
388.9	22.56	764.1	17.28
3.3	17.65	66.4	10.48
0.5	9.96	54.6	9.20
385.6	22.60	697.7	17.97
20.7	19.18	48.7	19.95
364.8	22.80	648.9	17.81
0.8	16.18	40.6	14.04
0.7	14.95	40.5	14.41
		1.1	10.00
66.1	12.94	154.6	13.34
66.1	12.94	154.1	13.31
5.9	8.10	24.9	7.79
0.3	4.43	273.6	10.86

trends in the economy. Thus, the overall number of jobs for child care workers plus preschool teachers is projected to grow about 13 percent over a decade from 2008 to 2018. Within that overall projection, preschool employment is projected to grow 19 percent and child care employment

11 percent. Wage and salary employment is projected to grow 16 percent, and self-employment only 5 percent. Similarly, child day care employment in centers is projected to grow by 12 percent, but employment in fitness and recreation centers by 14 percent. The greatest projected growth—22 percent—is for child care workers in the educational services sector; employment of preschool teachers in educational establishments is projected to grow by 10 percent.

These are of course projections, and changes in economic trends, professional practice, or public policies could yield different results. Because the classification that differentiates child care workers from preschool teachers is not consistent with current professional concepts in the field of early care and education, the differences between these two occupations are likely to vary.

Injuries and Illnesses Involved in Missing at Least One Day of Work[4]

The annual rate of illnesses and injuries for child care services (including workers responsible for school-aged children) is somewhat higher than the national average (115 per 10,000 full-time workers versus 106 for all U.S. workers). The child care rate is much higher than that for elementary–secondary education (115 vs. 60 per 10,000 workers).

The rate of illness and injury for child care services has increased in the last 2–3 years, while the overall national rate has not, and the educational services rate has declined. However, the year-to-year variability may be due to reflecting a relatively small sample of child care workers. BLS staff has advised us that the data cannot be averaged across years to provide a more stable estimate.

CHARACTERISTICS OF THE ECCE WORKFORCE

We compiled data regarding the characteristics of the ECCE workforce from the 50 studies described above and describe the workforce using these characteristics and the relative study rankings. In this summary we gave preference to studies based upon their (1) representativeness of the population, (2) coverage of the ECCE workforce, and (3) year of data collection. Thus, the contents of each of the tables in this report are primarily based upon the second set of studies (II). These studies are nationally representative, include most child care settings (except FFN), cover all B–5 caregivers, but do not distinguish them from caregivers of

---

[4] U.S. Bureau of Labor Statistics (BLS) runs provided 02-13-11. Occupational injury and illness data from the BLS Occupational Safety and Health Statistics program. Program information available at http://www.bls.gov/iif/.

school-aged children because they use Census occupational and industry codes.

We have added to these studies relevant data from two Census sources—the 2009 ACS and the 2010 CPS, which were specially tabulated for this study by the U.S. Bureau of Labor Statistics.[5] These tabulations reflect application of the occupation and industry codes cited here.

The occupations used in these analyses are based on the two following broad federal occupational codes:

- 2300: Preschool and kindergarten teachers
- 4600: Child care workers

The industries used in these analyses are based on the two following federal industry codes:

- 8470: Child day care services
- 9290: Private households (broader Census code that includes FCC providers)

Thus, the data reflect a somewhat broader workforce definition than the B–5 focus of the ECCE committee, because child care workers (4600) include care for school-aged children and the private households industry code (9290) includes other household workers beyond FCC providers. However, they do not include the sizeable FFN component, because most FFN caregivers do not identify themselves as in the child care occupation. When data are not available from this set of studies, we use additional studies reviewed for this report.

The first column of each table indicates the type and study ranking (I–VII) and the number of studies in this type. The additional columns provide estimates for child care providers, preschool teachers, directors, and FCC providers. The child care worker data in the first column of each table do not necessarily reflect the specific total of the characteristics by position (child care worker, preschool teacher, or FCC provider). Rather, they are independent estimates calculated by the cited studies for U.S. Census occupational codes. In some cases we report the combination of preschool and kindergarten teachers, because Census data do not distinguish these categories. From BLS data, which do use this distinction, we know that about two-thirds of the combined category is preschool

---

[5] U.S. Department of Labor, U.S. Bureau of Labor Statistics. Previously unpublished tabulations from the CPS (2010) and ACS (2009) conducted by the U.S. Census Bureau. These tabulations were from the PUMS files, which are a sample of the full microdata set. Personal communication with Dixie Sommers, assistant commissioner, February 11, 2011.

teachers, so the combined data are more reflective of preschool than kindergarten teachers.

Characteristics are divided into seven major areas:

1. *Demographic characteristics*: age, gender, race/ethnicity, marital status, and household composition and income
2. *Qualifications*: educational attainment, general and early childhood education (ECE)-specific, ECE experience, and bi- or multilingual communication
3. *Professional development*: training and credentials
4. *Labor market characteristics*: full-/part-time employment, hours worked per week, other employment
5. *Compensation*: wages, benefits
6. *Staff stability*: occupational and job turnover
7. *Professional status*: attitudes and orientation: union and professional organization membership

We describe each set of these characteristics below and present more detailed summaries of the studies included in a later section of this report. Detailed tables of characteristics of the ECCE workforce are available at http://www.iom.edu/Reports/2011/The-Early-Childhood-Care-and-Education-Workforce-Challenges-and-Opportunities.aspx.

Demographic Characteristics: Age, Gender, Race/Ethnicity, Marital Status, Household Composition and Income

Age of Workers

According to previously unpublished tabulations based on data from the CPS and the ACS, the median age for child care workers ranges from 35 to 39 years. The median age for preschool teachers is 39 years, but the median age for workers employed in private households, which include FCC providers, is higher—43 years.

The share of the workforce that may be considered adolescent babysitters has been an issue of interest. Across the studies, the percentage of caregivers under age 20 ranges from 5 to 9 percent. The percentage is highest for FCCs (about 7 percent) and lower for preschool teachers (<2 percent). The percentage of caregivers aged 65 years or older is also small, ranging from 4 to 5 percent. Table B-4 shows the median age of ECCE workers.

TABLE B-4 Median Age of Workers, 2009–2010

Type and N Studies	Child Care Workers	Preschool and Kindergarten Teachers*	FCC Providers
(II) 3	35–39	39	43

NOTE: FCC: Family Child Care.
* Census categories combine preschool and kindergarten teachers.
SOURCES: Unpublished tabulations of data from the CPS (2010) and the ACS (2009). U.S. Bureau of Labor Statistics, February 2011.

TABLE B-5 Percentage Female in Workforce, 2009–2010

Type and N Studies	Child Care Workers	Preschool and Kindergarten Teachers	FCC Providers
(II) 5	94.2–95.2	97.0–97.9	90.9–91.0

NOTE: FCC: Family Child Care. Data in this table reflect standard federal occupational and industry codes. Groups are not subsets of each other.
SOURCE: Unpublished tabulations of data from the CPS (2010) and the ACS (2009). U.S. Bureau of Labor Statistics, February 2011.

Gender

As shown in Table B-5, about 95 percent of the ECCE workforce is female. The percentage of women is highest for preschool and kindergarten teachers (97 percent).

Race/Ethnicity

Table B-6 shows data regarding the race and ethnicity of ECCE workers. The child care workforce is predominately white and non-Hispanic, with estimates ranging from 71 to 79 percent white for child care workers, 76 to 83 percent for preschool teachers, and 69 to 86 percent for FCC providers. A large minority of FCC providers (36 to 40 percent) are of Hispanic origin.

Additional comparisons of the race and ethnicity of child care workers with children age B–5 are available from the HSPC demand-based estimates study (Brandon et al., 2011), which used data from the ATUS. However, this summary does not include preschool teachers because they are not included in the Census occupational code for child care workers

TABLE B-6 Race/Ethnicity of Workers, 2009–2010

	Type and N Studies	Child Care Workers	Preschool and Kindergarten Teachers	FCC Providers
White, non-Hispanic (%)	(II) 5	70.5–78.6	75.6–82.7	69.3–85.5
African American, non-Hispanic (%)	(II) 5	15.8–18.0	13.4–16.5	8.7–10.1
Hispanic/Latina (%)	(II) 5	16.2–19.1	9.6–11.4	35.5–39.5
American Indian or Alaska Native (%)	(III) 2		0.9 (1997)–1.2 (2006)	
Asian or Pacific Islander (%)	(II) 2	2.6–2.9	2.2	3.4
Multiracial/biracial, other (%)	(II) 5	5.0–10.4	3.9–5.7	5.9–17.2

NOTE: FCC: Family Child Care. CPS and ACS data in this table reflect standard federal occupational and industry codes. Groups are not subsets of each other.
SOURCE: Except for estimates for percentage American Indian or Alaskan Native, which come from the Head Start FACES, data come from unpublished tabulations of data from the CPS (2010) and the ACS (2009). U.S. Bureau of Labor Statistics, February 2011.

and could not be distinguished from kindergarten teachers.[6] As Table B-7 shows, when averaging data from 2005 through 2007, the estimates for the race/ethnicity of child care workers are similar to those above. The percentage of child care workers who are white (75.9 percent) is very close to the percentage of children ages B–5 who are white (76.5 percent). However, there are some small differences in the percentage of workers and children who describe their racial group as black, other, and Hispanic. Averaging data from 2005 through 2007, 17.4 percent of child care workers identified as black, 6.7 percent as a racial group not listed (other), and 17.8 percent as Hispanic. In the same time period, 14.8 percent of children ages B–5 were identified as black, 8.8 percent as other, and 22.3 percentage as Hispanic. The large percentage of young children who were Hispanic reflects the growing Hispanic population in the United States. It is possible that this summary overstates the share of the ECCE workforce from

---

[6] Within the ATUS sample, 343 respondents (318 females and 25 males) listed their industry or occupation as child care worker. The industry code used for this analysis was 8470—child care day services—and the occupation code was 4600—child care workers. This sample is restricted to employed persons, but it did not have any other restrictions. This study did not use industry or occupation codes to define FFN caregivers. Caregiving was based on time spent in non-household childcare activities.

TABLE B-7 Race/Ethnicity for Child Care Workers and Children, 2005–2007 Average

Child Care Workers		Children Ages Birth–5	
	Percent		Percent
White	75.9	White	76.5
Black	17.4	Black	14.8
Other	6.7	Other	8.8
Hispanic	17.8	Hispanic	22.3

SOURCE: HSPC demand-based estimates. Brandon et al., 2011.

minority groups. That is because the non-included preschool teachers are likely to have a greater share of white and smaller share of other racial/ ethnic backgrounds, because they often have higher formal education requirements, and the rate of college attendance is substantially higher for whites.

Marital Status

Almost half (48 percent) of the total child care workers are married, with another third (33 percent) that have never been married, and almost a fifth (18 percent) who indicate that they are separated, widowed, or divorced, as shown in Table B-8.

Household Composition and Income

About two-thirds of child care workers have children present in their homes. A minority live alone (16–22 percent) or live with their parents (19–24 percent). The mean household income for a child care worker in 1993 was $26,835, which translates to approximately $40,495 in 2010 dollars. The mean household income for a preschool teacher in 2004 was

TABLE B-8 Marital Status of Child Care Workers, 2007

	Type and N Studies	Child Care Workers
Married (%)	(II) 1	48.3
Never married (%)	(II) 1	33.3
Formerly married (%)	(II) 1	18.4

SOURCE: HSPC demand-based estimates. Brandon et al., 2011.

TABLE B-9   Household Composition and Income

	Type and N Studies	Child Care Workers	Preschool Teachers
Children present in household (%)	(II) 1	68.3 (2007)	
Mean household income (dollars)	(III) 1; (IV) 1	26,835 (1993)	58,388 (2004)
Median household income (dollars)	(III) 1		52,000 (2004)

SOURCE: Estimates for the percentage child care workers with children present come from HSPC demand-based estimates. Brandon et al., 2011. Estimates for the mean household income of child care workers come from the CQCO, 1993. All other estimates come from the NPS, 2004.

$58,388, which translates to $67,579 in 2010 dollars. The median household income in 2004 was $52,000, which is equivalent to $60,185 in 2010 dollars. These data are presented in Table B-9.

The estimates for prekindergarten teachers in this table come from the NPS, which only sampled teachers of 3–4-year-olds. Preschool and prekindergarten teachers have higher compensation than other child care workers, and are therefore likely to have higher family incomes. It should be noted that 30 percent had incomes that are considered to be below the criterion for self-sufficiency, which is below twice the federal poverty level.

Qualifications: Educational Attainment—General and ECE-Specific, Professional Development, ECCE Experience, and Bi- or Multilingual Communication

Many of the studies we reviewed focused on assessing child care workers' qualifications and subsequently determining whether qualifications were correlated with quality of care. For this reason, there is a large amount of information on education attainment, early care and education training, and other types of professional development on the national and state level. However, few of the national studies, except those focused on preschool, restricted their samples to child care workers for B–5 children. The estimates summarized in Table B-10A come from provided tabulations of Current Population Survey data, which includes caregivers for school-aged children. The estimates summarized in Table B-10B come from the FACES studies and the MSSPK and SWEEP studies that only focused on prekindergarten teachers.

TABLE B-10A Educational Attainment, 2009–2010

	Type and N Studies	Child Care Workers	FCC Providers
a. High school diploma or equivalent (%)	(II) 6	26.7–33.2	32.2–33.4
b. Some college (%)	(II) 5	21.4–39.0	17.3–32.0
c. Associate's degree (%)	(II) 6	7.3–12.1	5.1–5.6
d. Bachelor's degree (%)	(II) 6	10.8–16.9	7.4–10.3
e. Graduate or professional degree (%)	(II) 5	1.9–4.4	1.2–2.0
f. Bachelor's degree or higher (%)	(II) 5	12.7–21.2	8.6–12.2

NOTES: FCC: Family Child Care. CPS and ACS data in this table come from occupational and industry codes. Groups are not subsets of each other.
SOURCES: Unpublished tabulations of data fromtthe CPS (2010) and the ACS (2009). U.S. Bureau of Labor Statistics, February 2011.

TABLE B-10B Educational Attainment, 2009–2010

	Type and N Studies	Preschool Teachers
a. High school diploma or equivalent (%)	(III) 5, (V) 2	2.0–22.0
b. Some college (%)	(III) 5, (V) 2	13.0–32.5
c. Associate's degree (%)	(III) 5, (V) 2	12.0–18.0
d. Bachelor's degree (%)	(V) 2	18.1–49.0
e. Graduate or professional degree (%)	(V) 2	24.0–25.6
f. Bachelor's degree or higher (%)	(III) 5, (V) 2	28.1–73.2

SOURCE: Data from (III) studies come from the Head Start FACES. Data from (V) study come from the MSSPK and the SWEEP.

Educational Attainment

Preschool teachers had the highest levels of educational attainment: 18 to 49 percent obtained a bachelor's degree, and 24 to 26 percent obtained a graduate or professional degree. However, preschool teachers in these studies come from samples based on state-sponsored programs, so it is likely that they have higher education levels than other prekindergarten teachers. Education levels were lower for child care workers and FCC providers. Approximately a third of each of these groups did not attend college past high school. However, 11 to 18 percent of child care workers

TABLE B-11 ECCE-Specific Education

	Type and N Studies	Preschool Teachers
Obtained associate's degree in ECE (%)	(V) 1	12 (2001)
Obtained bachelor's degree in ECE (%)	(III) 1, (V) 1	31 (2001)
Obtained advanced degree in ECE (%)	(IV) 1, (V) 1	13 (2001)
Obtained CDA (%)	(I) 1, (III) 7	22.8 (2004)–76.1 (1997)
Obtained a state awarded certificate (%)	(III) 2	29.3 (2004)–57.2 (2006)
Obtained a teaching certificate/license (%)	(III) 3	34 (2000)–38.6 (2006)

NOTE: CDA: Child Development Associate.
SOURCE: Data from (III) studies come from the Head Start FACES. Data from (V) study come from the MMSSPK and the SWEEP.

and 7 to 10 percent of FCC providers completed college with a bachelor's degree.

ECE-Specific Education

Caregivers and teachers vary in the amount of ECE-specific education that they obtained, as shown in Table B-11. As of 2001, 12 percent of preschool teachers had obtained an associate's degree in ECE, 31 percent obtained a bachelor's in ECE, and 13 percent obtained an advanced degree in ECE. The percentage of prekindergarten teachers who obtained a child development associate (CDA) credential, state-awarded certificate, or other type of teaching certificate varied across studies. For example, 23 percent of teachers in the 2004 National Prekindergarten Study had obtained a CDA, but 76 percent of teachers in the 1997 Head Start Family and Child Experiences Survey reported obtaining one.

Professional Development

Several studies also recorded whether teachers engaged in other types of professional development. Teachers in the National Prekindergarten Study spent an average of 33 hours in training within the past year, while 39 to 47 percent of teachers in the different waves of the Head Start Family and Child Experiences Survey were currently enrolled in teacher-related training at the time of the survey. These data are presented in Table B-12.

TABLE B-12 Professional Development

	Type and N Studies	Preschool Teachers
Mean hours in training in past 12 months (hours)	(III) 1	32.9 (2004)
Currently enrolled in teacher-related training (%)	(III) 3	38.7 (2006)–46.5 (2001)

SOURCE: 2004 data come from the NPS. 2001 and 2006 data come from the Head Start FACES.

TABLE B-13 Mean Years in Caregiving Field

Type and N Studies	Child Care Workers	Preschool Teachers
(I) 1, (III) 3, (V) 4	4.0–5.4 (1994)	6.8 (1997)–11.8 (2000)

SOURCES: 1994 data come from the NICHD SECCYD. 1997 data come from the NCEDL-S. 2000 data come from the Head Start FACES.

ECCE Experience

Across studies, child care workers reported having an average of 4 to 5 years of work experience in the ECCE field, while preschool teachers had an average of 7 to 12 years of experience. Head Start teachers had spent an average of 8 to 9 years teaching in Head Start classrooms.

Note that these data, shown in Table B-13, are estimates of current level of experience, not of the duration of time workers will remain in the field. They reflect questions asked of active workers, rather than of workers who had retired or left the field. The respondents would thus continue to work in the field for an underdetermined amount of time. Duration or tenure will thus exceed current years of experience, but we do not currently have data reflecting duration.

Labor Market Characteristics: Compensation (Wages, Benefits), Full-/Part-Time Employment, Hours Worked per Week, Other Employment, and Job and Occupational Turnover

Compensation

In this section we address two components of compensation: earnings and benefits (health and retirement).

Earnings The Bureau of Labor Statistics and the Current Population Survey provide median weekly earnings estimates for workers by occu-

TABLE B-14 Median Weekly Earnings (Dollars)

Type and N Studies	Child Care Workers	Preschool and Kindergarten Teachers	FCC Providers
(II) 2	400.00 (2010)	621.00 (2010)	269.23 (2010)

NOTE: FCC: Family Child Care. Data in this table reflect standard occupational and industry codes. Groups are not subsets of each other.
SOURCE: Child Care Worker and Preschool/Kindergarten Teacher data from the BLS (ftp://ftp.bls.gov/pub/special.requests/lf/aat39.txt). FCC studies based on unpublished tabulations of data from the CPS (2010), U.S. Bureau of Labor Statistics, February 2011.

pation and industry, which we include as our primary compensation estimates. As seen in Table B-14, child care workers earned an average of $400 per week in 2010, preschool and kindergarten teachers averaged $621 per week, and FCC providers earned the least—$269 per week.

As a point of comparison, for full-time, year-round workers, these median annual earnings would be approximately $20,800 for child care workers, $32,292 for teachers, and $14,000 for FCC providers if we were to multiply these estimates by 52 weeks in a year. By contrast, the median weekly wage across occupations in 2010 was $747 (or $38,844 annually).[7] However, many ECCE staff are not employed full-time and do not work at their jobs for 12 months a year. As shown in Table B-15, less than half of FCC providers work full-time, and at most two-thirds of child care workers are employed full-time. Because of the lack of full-time employment for ECCE workers, the yearly earnings estimates will be lower than those provided for full-time, year-round workers.

Many child care workers are also employed in school-based or school-related programs, which only operate about 9 months of the year. Enrollment at community-based child care centers drops substantially in the summer as parents take vacations and move houses; some staff takes vacation, others are temporarily not employed. However, even though they are not working at their normal ECCE jobs, such staff may be employed in other occupations or locations. Some teachers are employed in summer sessions. Others may use the time to gain college credits, which can increase their earnings. Therefore, the net financial impact of compensation for individual workers for varying employment throughout the year is not fully captured by any standard data source that we are aware of.

---

[7] U.S. Bureau of Labor Statistics, 2010, "Table 39: Median weekly earnings of full-time wage and salary workers by detailed occupation and sex," *Household Data Annual Averages*, ftp://ftp.bls.gov/pub/special.requests/lf/aat39.txt.

TABLE B-15 Percentage Who Work Full Time, 2009–2010

Type and N Studies	Child Care Workers	Preschool and Kindergarten Teachers	FCC Providers
(II) 4	51.0–64.7	71.3–74.2	37.8–42.6

NOTE: FCC: Family Child Care. Data in this table reflect standard federal occupational and industry codes. Groups are not subsets of each other.
SOURCE: Unpublished tabulations of data from the CPS (2010) and the ACS (2009). U.S. Bureau of Labor Statistics, February 2011; HSPC demand-based estimates. Brandon et al. (2011).

Weekly Hours and Full-Time/Part-Time Status

As shown in Table B-15, a large majority of the ECCE workforce, with the exception of FCC providers, worked full-time and many worked more than 40 hours per week. Preschool and kindergarten teachers as a group had the largest percentage of full-time workers (71–74 percent), child care workers (51–65 percent), and finally FCC providers (38–43 percent). These rates of full-time employment are all lower than the average for the total population of employed persons age 16 and older, which was approximately 80.3 percent in 2010.[8]

According to 2003–2007 data from the ATUS, child care workers reported working 34 hours per week on average; however in the BLS current employment series, employers report an average of 30.3 hours/week for child care workers. Teachers in the National Prekindergarten Study reported 37 hours per week of work. Teachers also reported spending an average of 4 hours per week in planning time for classes. About half of prekindergarten teachers (54 percent) performed 2 to 4 hours per week of unpaid planning time as well.

Benefits A major economic consideration for ECCE workforce is access to retirement and health benefits. In this section we summarize previously unpublished data from the 2010 National Compensation Survey provided specifically for this study.[9] As for other BLS data, we note that Child Care Workers and Child Day Care Services includes school-aged as well as ECCE workers. It should also be noted that the data do not distinguish between full- and part-time workers. Because part-time workers often

---

[8] Bureau of Labor Statistics, 2010, "Table 8: Employed and unemployed full- and part-time workers by age, sex, race, and Hispanic or Latino ethnicity," *Household Data Annual Averages*, ftp://ftp.bls.gov/pub/special.requests/lf/aat8.txt.

[9] U.S. Department of Labor, U.S. Bureau of Labor Statistics, Health and Retirement Benefit Access and Participation; Employer Costs for Employee Compensation, March 2010. Breakdown by selected occupations and industries. Personal communication with Philip M. Doyle, assistant commissioner, May 10, 2011.

receive fewer benefits, and the share of part-time workers is higher for ECCE than for the total population of civilian workers; the comparison between ECCE and total workers may be slightly overstated.

Tables B-16A through B-16F summarize employer-reported benefits for the two major components of the ECCE workforce regularly tracked by BLS: child care workers and preschool teachers. These are divided by the category of the establishment where they work: child day care services (column 2) versus elementary and secondary schools (column 3). Other workers in these establishments, such as directors or food service workers, are reflected in the first row—all workers—under the establishment category. Child care workers and preschool teachers in other types of establishments—e.g., health facilities—are reflected in rows 2–4 of the first column. For sake of comparison, the entry in the first row and first column shows the value for all civilian workers in all industries. It should be noted that the total includes the ECCE workers, but because they represent less than 1 percent (about 0.006) of the total workforce the error in the comparison is slight.

Health Benefits Table B-16A shows the share of child care and preschool workers with access to employer health benefits. Access for ECCE is slightly more than half the rate for all civilian employees: 38 versus 74 percent. Preschool teachers slightly exceed the national average, with 75

TABLE B-16A Percentage of Civilian Workers with Access to Employer-Provided Health Insurance

	All Industries	Child Day Care Services	Elementary and Secondary Schools	Child Day Care Services and Elementary and Secondary Schools
All workers (in all occupations)	74	49	88	84
Child care workers and preschool teachers, except special education	38	31	60	39
Child care workers	31	26	47	31
Preschool teachers, except special education	63	64	90	75

SOURCE: BLS National Compensation Survey, 2010.

TABLE B-16B Percentage of Civilian Workers Participating in Employer-Provided Health Insurance

	All Industries	Child Day Care Services	Elementary and Secondary Schools	Child Day Care Services and Elementary and Secondary Schools
All workers (in all occupations)	60	26	75	70
Child care workers and preschool teachers, except special education	22	12	44	20
Child care workers	16	9	37	15
Preschool teachers, except special education	43	29	60	43

SOURCE: BLS National Compensation Survey, 2010.

percent access having access to benefits. However, only 39 percent of child care workers have access.

Access varies greatly between workers in the community-based child day care services industry, for which access is 31 percent, and elementary-secondary schools, which have 60 percent access. Even within the schools, 90 percent of preschool teachers have access to health benefits, compared to 47 percent of child care workers. In child day care services, the rates are lower but the discrepancy just as great: 64 percent of preschool teachers have access versus 26 percent of child care workers.

However, not all employees participate in employer-sponsored plans to which they have access. For some, the contributions or co-payments may be too high. Others may be covered under their spouse or partner's plan. Table B-16B shows the actual participation.

Thus, while 38 percent of all ECCE employees have access to health benefits, only 58 percent of those actually participate. For child care workers, the take-up rate is only 53 percent yielding 16 percent with employer coverage, while for preschool teachers it is 68 percent, yielding 43 percent participation.

Just as there are discrepancies in the percentage of workers having access to and participating in health benefits, there appear to be discrepancies in the amount contributed by employers to those benefits. It should be noted that the average cost includes hours worked by part-time

TABLE B-16C Average Hourly Cost to Employers per Worker Participating in Employer-Provided Health Insurance: Author's Estimates

	All Industries	Child Day Care Services	Elementary and Secondary Schools	Child Day Care Services and Elementary and Secondary Schools
All workers (in all occupations)	3.06	1.30	5.62	5.30
Child care workers and preschool teachers, except special education	2.05	0.95	4.48	2.26
Child care workers	1.83	0.67	4.15	1.95
Preschool teachers, except special education	2.90	2.38	5.09	3.71

SOURCE: BLS National Compensation Survey, 2010.

employees who are likely to have fewer benefits. However, to the extent that ECCE employs a higher share of part-time employees than the overall civilian economy reflects part of the structural difference in employment and compensation.

Table B-16C shows that average hourly employer costs for ECCE are about one-third lower than for the average workers—$2.05 versus $3.06 per hour. The distribution within ECCE parallels that for access and participation. Employer costs for preschool teachers schools are close to the overall average—$2.90 versus $3.06. For those in elementary and secondary schools, the costs are close to that for all school employees—$5.09 versus $5.62 per hour.

Retirement Benefits Tables B-16D, B-16E, and B-16F show similar information regarding employer-based retirement benefits. While 69 percent of employees in all industries have access to retirement benefits, only 30 percent of child care workers and 47 percent of preschool teachers have such access. As with health benefits, access is much higher for workers in schools than in other facilities.

Of the 69 percent of all workers with access to retirement benefits, 55 percent participate. For child care workers, 18 percent out of the 30 percent with access participate, and for preschool teachers all of the 47 percent with access participate. Combining all ECCE workers—child care

TABLE B-16D Percentage of Civilian Workers with Access to Employer-Provided Retirement Benefits

	All Industries	Child Day Care Services	Elementary and Secondary Schools	Child Day Care Services and Elementary and Secondary Schools
All workers (in all occupations)	69	30	90	84
Child care workers and preschool teachers, except special education	34	18	67	31
Child care workers	30	—	64	27
Preschool teachers, except special education	47	—	74	49

NOTE: Dashes indicate no workers in this category or data did not meet publication criteria.
SOURCE: BLS National Compensation Survey, 2010.

TABLE B-16E Percentage of Civilian Workers Participating in Employer-Provided Retirement Plans

	All Industries	Child Day Care Services	Elementary and Secondary Schools	Child Day Care Services and Elementary and Secondary Schools
All workers (in all occupations)	55	21	87	80
Child care workers and preschool teachers, except special education	24	9	59	23
Child care workers	18	—	54	17
Preschool teachers, except special education	47	—	72	48

NOTE: Dashes indicate no workers in this category or data did not meet publication criteria.
SOURCE: BLS National Compensation Survey, 2010.

TABLE B-16F Average Hourly Cost to Employers per Worker Participating in Employer-Provided Retirement Benefits: Author's Estimates

	All Industries	Child Day Care Services	Elementary and Secondary Schools	Child Day Care Services and Elementary and Secondary Schools
All workers (in all occupations)	1.65	0.27	3.32	3.05
Child care workers and preschool teachers, except special education	0.75	0.13	1.85	0.70
Child care workers	0.48	—	1.45	0.49
Preschool teachers, except special education	1.41	—	2.69	1.42

NOTE: Dashes indicate that no workers in this category or data did not meet publication criteria.
SOURCE: BLS National Compensation Survey, 2010.

and preschool, community-based and schools—23 percent actually participate in retirement benefits out of the 31 percent who have access.

Table B-16F shows the average hourly employer contribution to employee retirement plans. The pattern is similar to that for health insurance. Child care workers have average benefits that are less than a third of the average worker—$0.48 versus $1.65—while preschool teachers' benefits are slightly lower. Benefits in schools are more generous than in community-based settings. Average retirement costs for all workers in schools are nearly double that for the average U.S. worker—$3.32 versus $1.65. Preschool teachers in schools receive about 20 percent lower retirement benefits—$2.69 per hour worked—which is still much higher than preschool teachers in non-school settings.

Other Employment

According to CPS data, a small percentage of child care workers (5 percent) also worked additional jobs outside of their main employment. Four percent of teachers and 3 percent of FCC providers had an additional job. Of those with additional employment, child care workers spent about

16 hours per week at an extra job and teachers spent about 15, according to the 1993 CQCO study. These data are presented in Table B-17.

Job and Occupational Turnover

Turnover is a concern for many researchers and policy makers in the child care field. It is important to distinguish between job turnover—changing jobs within the ECCE field—and occupational turnover—leaving ECCE for another field. National studies have generally showed annual job turnover rates to be about one-third of child care workers and 19 to 39 percent of teachers. Data from California, gathered as part of the 1994–2000 study, *Then and Now: Changes in Childcare Staffing*, indicate that job turnover between 1999 and 2000 for all teaching staff was about 32 percent and occupational turnover was about 16 percent. Teachers and staff in this study also experienced a 2 to 6 percent decrease in wages in this time period. Data on annual job turnover are presented in Table B-18.

Professional Attitudes and Orientation: Union and Professional Organization Membership

Various aspects of professionalism have been demonstrated to predict the observed quality of caregiving and child outcomes. We do not have reliable national data on attitudes and orientation. However, there are

TABLE B-17 Percentage of Workers With Additional Job, 2010

Type and N Studies	Child Care Workers	Preschool and Kindergarten Teachers	FCC Providers
(II) 2	5.1	4.1	3.3

NOTE: FCC: Family Child Care. Data in this table reflect standard federal occupational and industry codes. Groups are not subsets of each other.
SOURCE: Unpublished tabulations of data from the CPS (2010) and the ACS (2009). U.S. Bureau of Labor Statistics, February 2011.

TABLE B-18 Annual Job Turnover (%)

Type and N Studies	Child Care Workers	Center-Based Teachers
(I) 1, (IV) 1	33–36.4 (1993)	19 (1990)–38.7 (1993)

SOURCE: Data from 1990 come from the PCCS study. Data from 1993 come from the CQCO study.

data regarding the aspects of professionalism involved in deciding to join a union or professional association.

As expected, union participation was highest among preschool teachers. Twenty-one percent of teachers indicated that they were union members (Table B-19). Rates of union membership were lower for child care workers (4–6 percent) and lowest for FCC providers (<1 percent).

Additionally, 53 to 62 percent of teachers and 14 percent of total child care workers indicated that they were members of one or more professional associations (Table B-20).

TABLE B-19 Percentage of Workers Unionized, 2010

Type and N Studies	Child Care Workers	Preschool and Kindergarten Teachers	FCC Providers
(II) 2	3.5–6.3	20.8	0.80

NOTE: FCC: Family Child Care. Data in this table reflect standard federal occupational and industry codes. Groups are not subsets of each other.
SOURCE: Unpublished tabulations of data from the CPS (2010) and the ACS (2009). U.S. Bureau of Labor Statistics, February 2011.

TABLE B-20 Percentage of Members of Professional Organization

Type and N Studies	Child Care Workers	Preschool Teachers
(III) 3, (IV) 1	14 (1988)	52.9 (1997)–62 (2000)

NOTE: Groups are not subsets of each other.
SOURCE: 1988 data come from the NCCSS. 1997 and 2000 data come from the Head Start FACES.

STUDY LIST

I. **Nationally representative; cover all children age B–5 (birth–age 5) and distinguish B–5 from school age; include most settings (2)**

   1. Profile of Child Care Settings (PCCS), 1990
   2. National Households Education Survey (NHES); Human Services Policy Center (HSPC)/Center for the Child Care Workforce (CCW) Child Care Workforce Estimates Study, 2005

II. **Nationally representative; include most settings; cover all B–5 but do not distinguish from school-age (7)**

   1. Current Population Survey (CPS), 2004
   2. CPS; Occupation, 2010
   3. CPS; Industry, 2010
   4. American Community Survey (ACS); Occupation, 2009
   5. ACS; Industry, 2009
   6. Quarterly Census of Employment and Wages (QCEW), 2009
   7. American Time Use Survey (ATUS); HSPC Estimating the Economic Value of Early Care and Education, 2005–2007

III. **Nationally representative; cover a portion of B–5 workforce or settings; e.g., prekindergarten, Head Start (7)**

   1. Head Start Impact Study (HSIS), 2002–2006
   2. Head Start: The Family and Child Experiences Survey (FACES), 2006–2007
   3. Head Start: FACES, 2001
   4. Head Start: FACES, 2000
   5. Head Start: FACES, 1997
   6. National Prekindergarten Study (NPS), 2003–2004
   7. National Center for Early Development and Learning Survey (NCEDL-S), 1997

IV. **Multistate; cover all of B–5 workforce by child age and setting (4)**

   1. National Child Care Staffing Study (NCCSS), 1988
   2. Cost, Quality and Child Outcomes in Child Care Centers (CQCO), 1993
   3. National Day Care Study (NDCS), 1976–1977
   4. National Day Care Home Study (NDCHS), 1980

V. Multistate; cover portion of B–5 workforce and settings; e.g., prekindergarten (5)

1. National Institute of Child Health and Human Development (NICHD) Study of Early Child Care and Youth Development (SECCYD), 15 Months
2. NICHD SECCYD, 24 Months
3. NICHD SECCYD, 36 Months
4. Multi-State Study of Pre-Kindergarten (MSSPK), 2001
5. Statewide Early Education Programs Survey (SWEEP), 2001–2003

VI. Single state: cover all B–5 workforce (21)

1. AZ: Survey of Arizona's Early Education Workforce, 2004
2. CA: California Early Care and Education Workforce Study—Family Child Care Survey, 2005
3. CA: California Early Care and Education Workforce Study—Center Survey, 2005
4. FL: Child Care Workforce Study, 2006
5. IL: Illinois Department of Human Services (IDHS) Illinois Salary and Staffing Survey of Licensed Child Care Facilities, 2008
6. IN: Survey of Teachers and Directors Working in Licensed Child Care Centers and Unlicensed Child Care Ministries, 2007
7. ME: Maine Child Care Market Rate and Workforce Study, 2002
8. MN: Child Care Workforce in Minnesota, 2006–2007
9. MN: Child Care Workforce in Minnesota, 2006–2007
10. MN: Child Care Workforce in Minnesota, 2006–2007
11. NYC: New York City Early Childhood Educators Survey, 2006
12. NC: North Carolina Child Care Workforce Survey, 2003
13. OH: Workforce Study of Ohio Early Childhood Centers, Ohio Department of Job and Family Services (ODJFS), 2005
14. OH: Workforce Study of Ohio Early Childhood Centers, Ohio Department of Education (ODE), 2005
15. PA: Early Care and Education Provider Survey, 2002
16. UT: Study of Childcare Workforce in Utah, 2006
17. VA: Childcare Workforce Study in Metro Richmond, Virginia, 2003
18. WI: Statewide Child Care Surveys, 1980
19. WI: Statewide Child Care Surveys, 1988
20. WI: Statewide Child Care Surveys, 1994
21. WI: Statewide Child Care Surveys, 2001

VII.   **Single state: cover portion of B–5 workforce and settings; e.g., prekindergarten (4)**

1. CA: Changes in Child Care Staffing Study, 2000
2. MA: Cost Quality (CQ) Center Study, 2000–2001
3. MA: CQ Public School Study, 2000–2001
4. MA: CQ FCCH Study, 2000–2001

DESCRIPTION

I.   Nationally Representative Studies; Cover All Children Age B–5 (Birth–Age 5) and Distinguish B–5 from School Age; Include Most Settings

National Household Education Survey, Early Childhood Supplement (NHES); Human Services Policy Center (HSPC)/Center for the Child Care Workforce (CCW) Child Care Workforce Estimates Study

- **Study Dates: 1999, 2005**
- **Agency:** HSPC; CCW
- Demand-based estimation of the early child care and education workforce
- Uses 1999 and 2005 data from the NHES to calculate estimates of child care workforce
- NHES is a large-scale, nationally representative survey that asks respondents questions about the hours spent in a variety of care arrangements in a typical week.
- The NHES is a random-digit-dial telephone survey of the general population, with 7,198 household respondents with children age B–5.
- Limitations:

  o Study itself does not sample ECCE workers.

Sources

Brandon, R. N., T. J. Stutman, and M. Maroto. 2011. The economic value of early care and education in the U.S. In *Economic Analysis: The Early Childhood Sector*, ed. E. Weiss and R. Brandon. Washington, DC: Partnership for America's Economic Success.

Center for the Child Care Workforce and Human Services Policy Center. 2002. *Estimating the size and components of the U.S. child care workforce and caregiving population: Key findings from the child care workforce estimate, executive summary: Preliminary report.* Washington, DC: Center for the Child Care Workforce.

Profile of Child Care Settings (PCCS)

- **Study Date: 1990**
- **Agency:** Mathematica Policy Research Group
- This study's goal was to focus on the availability (supply side) of early education care.
- The study is a nationally representative sample drawn from the universe of formal early education care programs.
- Computer-assisted telephone interviewing (CATI) survey with nationally representative sample of center directors and regulated home-based child care providers that are licensed or registered by the state or county in which they are located.
- Uses a two-stage clustered sample design: (1) 100 representative counties stratified according to region, metro status, and poverty level and (2) centers within counties.
- **Sample N:** 2,089 centers and 583 regulated home-based child care providers
- Provide weighted estimates in report
- Limitations:

  o Year/age of study

Source

Kisker, E. E., S. L. Hofferth, D. A. Phillips, and E. Farquhar. 1991. *A profile of child care settings: Early education and care in 1990.* Princeton, NJ: Mathematica Policy Research, Inc.; Washington, DC: Department of Education.

II. Nationally Representative; Most Settings; Cover All B–5 But Do Not Distinguish from School-Age

American Community Survey (ACS)

- **Data Date: 2009 single-year estimates**
- **Agency:** U.S. Census Bureau
- The ACS is a nationally representative survey based on housing units, with an additional survey for those persons living in group quarters.
- The ACS uses monthly samples to produce annual data for the same small areas (census tracts and block groups) formerly surveyed via the decennial census long-form sample.
- The Public Use Microdata Sample (PUMS) files contain records for a subsample of ACS housing units and group quarters persons, with information on the characteristics of these housing

units and group quarters persons plus the people in the selected housing units.
- The ACS produces 1-year, 3-year, and 5-year samples; this project utilizes the 1-year samples.
- Tabulations from PUMS data:

  o 2009 ACS demographics for Current Population Survey (CPS) aggregations of ECCE occupations, all detailed ECCE industries
  o Industries: elementary and secondary school, child day care services, private households

- Limitations:

  o Estimates are based on Census industry and occupation codes, which are not restricted to ECCE caregivers. They may include caregivers for school-aged children as well.
  o Industry codes also not specific to child care workers

American Time Use Survey (ATUS); HSPC Estimating the Economic Value of Early Care and Education

- **Study Dates: 2005–2007**
- **Agency:** HSPC (analysis); Bureau of Labor Statistics (BLS) (data)
- Provides characteristics of child care workers from the ATUS
- The ATUS is conducted by the BLS and administered by the U.S. Census. Surveyors randomly select individuals from a subset of households from the CPS and interview these respondents about how they spent their time on the previous day, where they were, and whom they were with.
- These estimates were calculated in relation to a project focused on hours of caregiving.
- **Sample N:** 501 child care workers
- Limitations:

  o Uses census categorization to define child care workers; therefore does not include preschool teachers and may include children of any age

Source
Brandon, R. N., T. J. Stutman, and M. Maroto. 2011. The economic value of early care and education in the U.S. In *Economic Analysis: The Early Childhood Sector*, ed. E. Weiss and R. Brandon. Washington, DC: Partnership for America's Economic Success.

Current Population Survey

- **Study Dates: 1979-2004; 2010**
- **Agency:** Economic Policy Institute (analysis); U.S. Census Bureau (data)
- CPS is a monthly survey of 60,000 U.S. households
- Study using 1979–2004 data (Herzenberg et al., 2005):

  o This study uses three different CPS extracts to produce numbers of child care workers based on educational attainment, wages, and benefits.
  o Estimates and characteristics about child care providers based on census occupation and industry codes

    ▪ 2000–2003 data: Industry Code = 8470 (child day-care services)
    ▪ 2000–2003 data: Occupation Code = 4600 (child care workers)

  o Data are provided for child care workers from 1979 through 2004

- Tabulations from PUMS data:

  o 2009 ACS and 2010 CPS demographics for CPS aggregations of ECCE occupations, all detailed ECCE industries
  o Occupations: education administrators, preschool and kindergarten teachers, special education teachers, teacher assistants, first line supervisors/managers, child care workers
  o Industry: elementary and secondary schools, child day care services, private households

- Limitations:

  o Estimates are based on Census industry and occupation codes, which are not restricted to ECCE caregivers. They may include caregivers for school-aged children as well.

Source

Herzenberg, S., M. Price, and D. Bradley. 2005. *Losing ground in early childhood education: Declining workforce qualifications in an expanding industry, 1979-2004.* Washington, DC: Economic Policy Institute.

Quarterly Census of Employment and Wages (QCEW)

- **Date: 2009**
- **Agency:** BLS; U.S. Department of Labor
- Near-census of monthly employment and quarterly wage information by six-digit North American Industry Classification System (NAICS) industry at the national, state, and county levels
- Limitations:

  o Estimates are based on Census industry and occupation codes, which are not restricted to ECCE caregivers. They may include caregivers for school-aged children as well

III. Nationally Representative; Cover a Portion of B–5 Workforce or Settings, e.g., Prekindergarten, Head Start

Head Start: The Family and Child Experiences Survey (FACES)

- **Study Waves/Dates: 1997–2001, 2000–2001, 2003–2004, 2006–2007**
- **Agency:** U.S. Department of Health and Human Services, Administration on Children, Youth and Families

  o http://www.acf.hhs.gov/programs/opre/hs/faces/

- This survey has multiple waves that are part of Head Start's Program Performance Measures Initiative.
- Each cohort survey of FACES employs a nationally representative sample of Head Start programs, centers, classrooms, children, and parents.
- The sample is stratified by region (Northeast, Midwest, South, West), urbanicity, and percentage of minority families in the program
- **2006–2007 Cohort:** National random sample of Head Start Programs from Head Start Program Information Report

  o Sample: 60 programs, 135 centers, 410 classroom, 365 teachers, 3,315 children (Fall 2006)

- **2003–2004 Cohort:** National random sample of Head Start Programs from Head Start Program Information Report (follow-up child sample)

  o Sample: 63 programs; 2,400 children

- **2000–2001 Cohort:** National random sample of Head Start Programs from Head Start Program Information Report (second sample)

  o Sample: 43 programs; 2,800 children; Fall 2000—257 teachers; Spring 2001—264 teachers

- **1997–2001 Cohort:** National random sample of Head Start Programs from Head Start Program Information Report (first sample)

  o First cohort with six phases

    ▪ Phase 1—field test of 2,400 children and parents in Spring 1997, Phases 2 and 3—survey interviews of 3,200 children and families and 437 teachers in Fall 1997; Phase 4—follow-up Spring 1999; Phase 5—follow-up Spring 2000; Phase 6—follow-up Spring 2001

  o Sample: 40 programs; 3,200 children and parents; 437 teachers

- Limitations:

  o Data are restricted to Head Start programs, centers, classrooms, children, and parents

Sources

Aikens, N., L. Tarullo, L. Hulsey, C. Ross, J. West, and Y. Xue. 2010. *ACF-OPRE report: A year in Head Start: Children, families, and programs*. Washington, DC: U.S. Department of Health and Human Services, Administration for Children and Families, Office of Planning, Research and Evaluation.

Hulsey, L., N. Aiken, Y. Xue, L. Tarullo, and J. West. 2010. *ACF-OPRE report: Data tables for FACES 2006 A Year in Head Start report*. Washington, DC: U.S. Department of Health and Human Services, Administration for Children and Families, Office of Planning, Research and Evaluation.

U.S. Department of Health and Human Services, Administration for Children and Families. 2006. *Head Start Performance Measures Center Family and Child Experiences Survey (FACES 2000) technical report*. Washington, DC: U.S. Department of Health and Human Services.

Head Start Impact Study (HSIS)

- **Study Dates: 2002–2006**
- **Agency:** U.S. Department of Health and Human Services, Administration on Children, Youth and Families

  o http://www.acf.hhs.gov/programs/opre/hs/impact_study/index.html

- **Sampling process:**

    o Identified grantee/delegate agencies using the Head Start Program Information Report (PIR) after excluding agencies that only serve special populations, those that were involved in the FACES study, and those that were "extremely new to the program" to create a list of 1,715 agencies;
    o Organized the list into 161 geographic clusters, then stratified it into 25 strata varying by region, location, race/ethnicity, policies, and other factors. Selected a cluster of programs from each of the 25 strata;
    o Determined eligibility of the agencies creating a pool of 223 agencies;
    o Grouped and stratified these along other regional conditions, to create a sample of 90 agencies across 23 states;
    o Agencies recruited and dropped 3;
    o Developed list of 1,427 Head Start Centers;
    o Determined eligibility of centers;
    o Re-stratified eligible centers;
    o Selected children and conducted random assignment

- **Sample N:** 2,783 Head Start children and 1,884 control children for total sample of 4,667 children
- Data collection included: direct child assessments, parent interviews, teacher surveys and child reports, center director setting interviews, and care setting observations
- Caregiver information collected:

    o Certificates, education, experience
    o Beliefs and attitudes

- Results are provided in terms of center setting for 3- and 4-year-old children in Head Start and control groups.
- Limitations:

    o Data are restricted to Head Start programs, centers, classrooms, children, and parents.

Source
U.S. Department of Health and Human Services, Administration for Children and Families. 2010. *Head Start Impact Study, final report*. Washington, DC.

National Center for Early Development and Learning (NCEDL) Survey

- **Study Dates: 1997**
- **Agency:** National Center for Early Development and Learning

  o http://www.fpg.unc.edu/~ncedl/

- The study consists of a stratified sample on eight levels of program type (national or local chain, independent for-profit, religious affiliate, Head Start, public school, independent nonprofit, other public agency, unknown) and four levels of program size (less than 40, 40-99, 100+children, unknown)
- **Sample Population:** Sample selected from a population of 85,715 early childhood programs provided in a list purchased from a commercial firm
- Mailed 4,979 surveys to a random stratified sample of the population
- **Sample N:** Final sample of 1,920 ECE teachers of 3- and 4-year-olds
- Directors filled out general questions about center; one teacher of 3–4-year-olds filled out the rest of the information.
- Limitations:

  o Sample restricted to teachers of 3–4-year-olds.
  o Sample does not include all B–5 teachers.

Source
Saluja, G., D. M. Early, and R. M. Clifford. 2002. Demographic characteristics of early childhood teachers and structural elements of early care and education in the United States. *Early Childhood Research and Practice* 4(1):1-19, http://ecrp.uiuc.edu/v4n1/saluja.html.

National Prekindergarten Study (NPS)

- **Study Dates: 2003–2004**
- **Agency:** Yale Child Study Center
- The study is a large-scale sample of prekindergarten teachers who had primary responsibility for a state-funded prekindergarten classroom.
- **Sample Population:** all 40,211 state-funded prekindergarten classrooms in the nation
- **Sample N:** National sample of 3,898 prekindergarten teachers
- Limitations:

  o Sample of prekindergarten teachers.
  o Sample does not include all B–5 ECE workers.

Source

Gilliam, W. S., and C. M. Marchesseault. 2005. *From capitols to classrooms, policies to practice: State-funded prekindergarten at the classroom level. Part 1: Who's teaching our youngest students? Teacher education and training, experience, compensation and benefits, and assistant teachers.* New Haven, CT: Yale University, Yale Child Study Center.

IV. Multistate; Cover All of B–5 Workforce by Child Age and Setting

Cost, Quality, and Child Outcomes in Child Care Centers

- **Study Dates: 1993–1994**
- **Agency:** University of Colorado, University of California, Los Angeles (UCLA), University of North Carolina at Chapel Hill, and Yale University
- This study examines the relationship between cost and quality of early childhood care and education programs in four states: California, Colorado, Connecticut, and North Carolina.
- The study uses a stratified random sample of 100 centers in each state (California, Colorado, Connecticut, and North Carolina).
- **Sample population:** Drew child care facilities from state-level lists of licensed child care facilities, excluded family child care programs, and only included early childhood programs that served infants, toddlers, and/or preschoolers.
- **Sample N:** 401 centers (200 for-profit and 201 non-profit), 228 infant/toddler classrooms, 521 preschool classrooms; 826 preschool children; 795 teachers
- Administrators of programs in the sampling area participated in telephone interviews, then if given permission, researchers collected data at each of the centers.
- Researchers observed classrooms at each center and collected most information about center and staff collected through a director interview.
- Additionally, all staff observed in classrooms also completed staff questionnaires that were adapted from the National Child Care Staffing Study.
- Limitations:

  o Multistate sample, not a random sample of the entire population
  o Date of study

Source

Helburn, S. W. 1995. *Cost, quality, and child outcomes in child care centers, technical report.* Denver, CO: University of Colorado, Department of Economics, Center for Research in Economic and Social Policy.

National Child Care Staffing Study (NCCSS)

- **Study Dates: 1988, 1992, and 1997**
- **Agency:** Center for Child Care Workforce

  o http://www.acf.hhs.gov/programs/opre/other_resrch/eval_
    data/reports/common_constructs/com_appb_nccss.html

- The study is based on a cross-section of 227 child care centers in Atlanta, Boston, Detroit, Phoenix, and Seattle.
- Five sites were chosen because they varied based on: level of quality required by each state in child care regulations, geographic region, relative distributions of for-profit and non-profit centers, and the attention accorded to child care staffing issues in state and local policy initiatives.

  o Three sites participated in the Cost Effects Study of the National Day Care Study in 1977 (Atlanta, Detroit, Seattle)

- Within each state pool of centers identified through lists of licensed child care centers

  o Pool within each state then divided into six groups: based on low-, middle-, and high-income tracts, and urban or suburban neighborhoods

- **1988 Sample N:** 643 classrooms with 1,309 teaching personnel, 865 teachers (805 teachers and 60 teacher/directors), 444 assistants (286 asst teachers and 158 aides)
- **1992 Sample N:** 193 centers, just re-interviewing directors
- **1997 Sample N:** 157 centers, just interviewing directors
- The study is not based on a national random sample, but does represent centers of varying population size, residential location, auspice, and quality.
- Data were collected through classroom observations and interviews with center directors and staff.
- Limitations:

  o Sample is not a national random sample
  o Multicity study

Sources

Whitebook, M., C. Howes, and D. Phillips. 1990. *Who cares? Child care teachers and the quality of care in America. Final report: National Child Care Staffing Study.* Oakland, CA: Child Care Employee Project.

Whitebook, M., D. Phillips, and C. Howes. 1993. *National Child Care Staffing Study revisited: Four years in the life of center-based care.* Oakland, CA: Child Care Employee Project.
Whitebook, M., C. Howes, and D. Phillips. 1998. *Worthy work, unlivable wages: The National Child Care Staffing Study, 1988-1997.* Oakland, CA: Child Care Employee Project.

National Day Care Study (NDCS)

- **Study Dates: 1976–1977**
- The study is a nationally representative survey of centers that restricted its coverage to centers operating at least 25 hours per week and 9 months per year, with a licensed capacity of 12 or more children and enrollments including 50 percent or fewer handicapped children.
- **Sample Population:** Centers selected from national lists constructed from state licensing lists

  o 18,307 centers with 897,700 children met selection criteria

- **Sample N:** 3,167 centers
- Limitations:

  o Year of study
  o Multi-state study

Source
Kisker, E. E., S. L. Hofferth, D. A. Phillips, and E. Farquhar. 1991. *A profile of child care settings: Early education and care in 1990.* Princeton, NJ: Mathematica Policy Research, Inc.; Washington, DC: Department of Education.

National Day Care Home Study (NDCHS)

- **Study Dates: 1976–1980**
- The study consists of a series of case studies of home-based care.
- The sample consists of both regulated and unregulated family day care homes in three urban areas (Los Angeles, Philadelphia, and San Antonio).
- **Sample N:** 793 family day care providers
- Limitations:

  o Year of study
  o Multistate study

Source
Kisker, E. E., S. L. Hofferth, D. A. Phillips, and E. Farquhar. 1991. *A profile of child care settings: Early education and care in 1990.* Princeton, NJ: Mathematica Policy Research, Inc.; Washington, DC: Department of Education.

V. Multistate; Cover Portion of B–5 Workforce and Settings; e.g., Prekindergarten

National Center for Early Development and Learning's Multi-State Pre-Kindergarten Study

- **Study Dates: 2001–2002 school year**
- **Agency:** NCEDL

  o http://www.fpg.unc.edu/~ncedl/
  o http://www.fpg.unc.edu/~ncedl/pages/pre-k_study.cfm

- The study is a stratified random sample of 237 lead teachers and 939 children in state-funded prekindergarten classrooms from six states (California, Georgia, Illinois, Kentucky, New York, and Ohio).
- **Sample Population:** The sample was drawn from a list of programs/centers provided by each state department of education.
- Researchers then stratified the sample in all states to maximize diversity with regard to teachers' education, program location, and program length.
- **Sample N:** 237 lead teachers and 939 children in state-funded prekindergarten classrooms from six states
- Limitations:

  o Sample restricted to teachers in state-funded prekindergarten classrooms from six states

Sources

Early, D. M., D. M. Bryant, R. C. Pianta, R. M. Clifford, M. R. Burchinal, S. Ritchie, C. Howesc, and O. Barbarin. 2006. Are teachers' education, major, and credentials related to classroom quality and children's academic gains in prekindergarten? *Early Childhood Research Quarterly* 21:174-195.

Pianta, R., C. Howes, M. Burchinal, D. Bryant, R. Clifford, D. Early, and O. Barbarin. 2005. Features of prekindergarten programs, classrooms, and teachers: Prediction of observed classroom quality and teacher-child interactions. *Applied Developmental Science* 9(3):144-159.

National Center for Early Development and Learning's Statewide Early Education Programs Survey (SWEEP)

- **Study Dates: 2003–2004 school year**
- **Agency:** NCEDL

  o http://www.fpg.unc.edu/~ncedl/pages/sweep.cfm

- This study is a stratified random sample of 465 lead teachers and 1,840 children in state-funded prekindergarten classrooms from five states (Massachusetts, New Jersey, Texas, Washington, and Wisconsin).
- **Sample Population:** The sample was drawn from a list of programs/centers provided by each state department of education.
- Researchers then stratified the sample in all states to maximize diversity with regard to teachers' education, program location, and program length.
- Prekindergarten programs in these five states were chosen because the states had models differing from those in the MSSPK study.
- **Sample N:** 465 lead teachers and 1,840 children in state-funded prekindergarten classrooms from five states
- Limitations:

   o Sample restricted to teachers in state-funded prekindergarten classrooms from five states

Source

Early, D., O. Barbarin, D. Bryant, M. Burchinal, F. Chang, R. Clifford, G. Crawford, W. Weaver, C. Howes, S. Ritchie, M. Kraft-Sayre, R. Pianta, and W. S. Barnett. 2005. *Prekindergarten in eleven states: NCEDL's multi-state study of pre-kindergarten and Study of State-Wide Early Education Programs (SWEEP): Preliminary descriptive report.* NCEDL Working Paper [combined results for Multi-State Pre-K Study and SWEEP]. Chapel Hill, NC: Frank Porter Graham Child Development Institute.

NICHD Study of Early Child Care and Youth Development (SECCYD)

- **Study Dates: Five phases from 1991–2007**
- **Agency:** National Institute of Child Health and Human Development, Early Child Care Research Network

   o http://www.nichd.nih.gov/research/supported/seccyd/overview.cfm

- Phase I, ages 0–3: 1991–1994 (1,364 children)
- Phase II, through 1st grade: 1995–1999 (1,226)
- Phase III, through 6th grade: 2000–2004 (1,061)
- Phase IV, through 9th grade: 2005–2007 (1,009)
- Caregivers of children in the study interviewed when children were at 15 months, 24 months, and 36 months

- **Sample N:** Caregivers for 1,216 children; 907 caregivers for 15-month-olds; 976 caregivers for 24-month-olds; 1,109 caregivers for 36-month-olds
- Limitations:

    o Sampling based on the children, not the caregivers

Sources

National Institute of Child Health and Human Development, Early Child Care Research Network. 1996. Characteristics of infant child care: Factors contributing to positive caregiving. *Early Childhood Research Quarterly* 11(3):269-306.

National Institute of Child Health and Human Development, Early Child Care Research Network. 2000. Characteristics and quality of child care for toddlers and preschoolers. *Applied Developmental Science* 4(3):116-135.

VI. Single State; Cover All B–5 Workforce

Arizona

Survey of Arizona's Early Education Workforce

- **Survey Dates: 1997, 2001, 2004**
- **Agency:** Arizona State Board on School Readiness, Governor's Office of Children, Youth, and Families, Association for Supportive Child Care, and Children's Action Alliance
- Telephone survey of all licensed early education employers in the state, excluding home-based businesses
- **Sample Population:** 2,117 licensed sites in September 2004 that provided care
- **Sample N:** 1,308 center administrators, 1,228 individual interviews in 2,142 programs
- Data are provided for teachers, assistant teachers, teacher directors, administrative directors

Source

Compensation and credentials: A survey of Arizona's early education workforce. 2005. Arizona State Board on School Readiness, Governor's Office of Children, Youth, and Families, Association for Supportive Child Care, and Children's Action Alliance, http://www.azchildren.org/MyFiles/PDF/CC_Compensation_Credentials.pdf.

California

California Early Care and Education Workforce Study

- **Study Date: 2005**

- **Agency:** Center for the Study of Child Care Employment and California Child Care Resource and Referral Network
- Statewide survey of CA licensed child care workforce
- **Survey Population:** Survey population included the 37,366 active licensed homes and 8,740 active licensed centers, serving children from birth to age 5, that were listed as of January 2004 with state-funded child care resource and referral agencies
- Statewide random sample of 1,800 licensed family child care homes and 1,921 centers, using a CATI system.
- **Sample N:** Center Survey

  o Sample population included 8,740 active licensed centers
  o 400 centers in four regions of the state
  o 1,921 total interviews with directors in centers that are licensed to care for children from birth to 23 months (infants) and/or from 2 to 5 years old and not yet in kindergarten (preschoolers)
  o Provide weighted estimates of the population of CA centers licensed to serve infants and/or preschoolers

- **Sample N:** FCC Survey

  o Survey population included all 37,366 of the active licensed family child care homes
  o 400 homes in four regions

Sources

Whitebook, M., L. Sakai, F. Kipnis, Y. Lee, D. Bellm, M. Almaraz, and P. Tran. 2006. *California Early Care and Education Workforce Study: Licensed child care centers. Statewide 2006.* Berkeley, CA: Center for the Study of Child Care Employment; San Francisco, CA: California Child Care Resource and Referral Network, http://www.irle.berkeley.edu/cscce/2006/california-early-care-and-education-workforce-study/.

Whitebook, M., L. Sakai, F. Kipnis, Y. Lee, D. Bellm, R. Speiglman, M. Almaraz, L. Stubbs, and P. Tran. 2006. *California Early Care and Education Workforce Study: Licensed family child care providers. Statewide 2006.* Berkeley, CA: Center for the Study of Child Care Employment; San Francisco, CA: California Child Care Resource and Referral Network.

Whitebook, M., F. Kipnis, and D. Bellm. 2008. *Diversity and stratification in California's early care and education workforce.* Berkeley, CA: Center for the Study of Child Care Employment, University of California.

Changes in Child Care Staffing Study

- **Study Dates: Three Waves, 1994, 1996, 2000**
- **Agency:** CCW
- This study focuses on staffing crisis in early childhood education and conducts a survey of caregivers in three areas of CA.

- Based in three Bay Area communities of Santa Cruz, San Mateo, and Santa Clara in Northern California
- Longitudinal study of center caregivers from 1994 through 2000
- Data come from interviews and classroom observations.
- **Sample Population:** NAEYC-accredited centers in three CA communities
- **Sample N 1994 and 1996:** 92 centers (observations and interviews in all), two preschool classrooms per center; 266 teaching staff observed in 1994; 260 staff observed in 1996

  o Generally classrooms serving 2.5- to 5-year-olds

- **Sample N 2000:** 75 centers (85 percent of 1996 sample), 43 observed, 32 interview-only, observed 117 teaching staff, 83 teachers, 20 assistants, 14 teacher-directors; 75 directors—interviews providing information about staff at the center
- Total staff at 75 centers: 435 teachers, 182 assistants, 42 teacher-directors

Source

Whitebook, M., L. Sakai, E. Gerber, and C. Howes. 2001. *Then and now: Changes in child care staffing, 1994-2000*. Berkeley, CA: Center for the Study of Child Care Employment; San Francisco, CA: California Child Care Resource and Referral Network.

Infrastructure Survey

- Non-random and not a complete census survey
- Online survey with SurveyMonkey
- 2009: surveyed a population of 1,588 persons who work in three types of early childhood infrastructure organizations in California—child care resource and referral programs, local First 5 commissions and as child care coordinators
- 1,091 completed interviews; 69 child care coordinators and staff, 285 First 5 staff, 737 R&R staff

Source

Whitebook, M. L., and F. Kipnis. 2010. *Beyond homes and centers: The workforce in three California early childhood infrastructure organizations*. Berkeley, CA: Center for the Study of Child Care Employment, Institute for Research on Labor and Employment, University of California, http://www.irle.berkeley.edu/cscce/wp-content/uploads/2010/08/beyond_homes_and_centers_es_100602-web-version.pdf.

Florida

Child Care Workforce Study

- **Study Date: 2006**
- **Agency:** Children's Forum, Inc.
- **Sample Population:** Beginning sample of 275 cases in May 2006, 136 child care centers (CCCs) and 139 family child care homes (FCCHs)

  o All centers were located in Seminole County, FL

- Surveyed entire population and adapted surveys from the CCW

  o 132 surveys returned, 88 CCCs and 44 FCCHs

- **Sample N:** 88 CCCs: 894 teachers, 334 assistant teachers, 71 teacher-directors, 94 directors (1,393 personnel)

Source
Esposito, B., and P. Kalifeh. 2006. *Child Care Workforce Study.* The Early Learning Coalition of Seminole and Children's Forum, Inc. http://www.fcforum.org/downloads/publications/Seminole%20WorkforceStudy%202006.pdf.

Illinois

Illinois Department of Human Services (IDHS) Illinois Salary and Staffing Survey of Licensed Child Care Facilities

- **Study Dates: 2007, 2009**
- **Agency:** IDHS
- **Sample Population:** all 13,953 facilities, 3,196 licensed child care centers and 10,757 licensed family child care home providers, who were listed in the Illinois Network of Child Care Resources & Referral Agencies (INCCRRA) database as providing care as of December 31, 2008
- **Sample N 2007:** 2007 sample of 13,467 licensed child care providers
- **Sample N 2009:** 2009 sample of 13,953 licensed child care providers
- Survey invitations were sent to all 13,953 facilities, 3,196 licensed child care centers and 10,757 licensed family child care home providers, who were listed in the INCCRRA database as providing care as of December 31, 2008.

- Of the 585 centers responding to the survey, 43 (7.14 percent) were completed by owners, 110 (18.27 percent) by owner/directors, 308 (51.16 percent) by directors, 72 (11.96 percent) by director/ teachers, and 52 (8.64 percent) by other personnel, including assistant/associate directors, human resources personnel, business/ fiscal personnel, executive directors, and site directors. Seventeen respondents did not report a title.

Sources

Garnier, P. C. 2008. *IDHS Illinois Salary and Staffing Survey of Licensed Child Care Facilities: FY2007.* Department of Human and Community Development, University of Illinois at Urbana-Champaign for the Illinois Department of Human Services, http://www.dhs. state.il.us/page.aspx?item=38614.

Wiley, A. R., S. King, and P. C. Garnier. 2009. *IDHS Illinois Salary and Staffing Survey of Licensed Child Care Facilities: FY2009.* Department of Human and Community Development, University of Illinois at Urbana-Champaign, http://www.dhs.state.il.us/page. aspx?item=49144.

Status of Early Childhood Workforce in Illinois, 2008

- Reports results of IDHS Illinois Salary and Staffing Survey with some added surveys
- Three statewide surveys: (1) 400 administrators of child care centers, (2) 800 lead teachers in community-based care and Head Start, (3) 150 teachers in public school settings

Source

Fowler, S., P. J. Bloom, T. Talan, S. Beneke, and R. Kelton. 2008. *Who's caring for the kids? The status of the early childhood workforce in Illinois.* Wheeling, IL: McCormick Tribune Center for Early Childhood Leadership, National-Louis University, and Early Childhood Parenting Collaborative, University of Illinois, http://cecl.nl.edu/research/reports/ whos_caring_report_2008.pdf.

Indiana

Survey of Teachers and Directors Working in Licensed Child Care Centers and Unlicensed Child Care Ministries

- **Study Date: 2007**
- **Agency:** Indiana Association for the Education of Young Children, Inc.
- Study consists of a mail survey in Indiana in 2007
- **Sample Population:** Originally mailed to all located centers: 1,235 directors and 14,834 teachers
- **Sample N:** Final response: 5,102 teachers and 668 directors

Source

Indiana Association for the Education of Young Children. 2007 *Working in child care in Indiana: 2007 special report on teachers and directors working in licensed child care centers and unlicensed registered child care ministries.* Indiana Association for the Education of Young Children, http://editor.ne16.com/iaeyc/2007_Workforce_Study_SpecialReport.pdf.

Iowa

Early Care and Education Workforce Study, 2003

- Little information about study design and sample in report

Source

Who's caring for Iowa's children: Early Care and Education Workforce Study 2003. Iowa Early Care & Education Professional Development Project, http://www.extension.iastate.edu/Publications/SP222.pdf.

Maine

Maine Child Care Market Rate and Workforce Study

- **Study Date: 2002**
- **Agency:** Mills Consulting Group, Inc.
- Two surveys, distributed by mail to all licensed child care centers (N = 712) and to all licensed family child care providers (N = 2054) using the Office of Child Care and Head Start licensing list
- **Sample Population:** all licensed centers and providers in Maine
- **Sample N:** 1,878 surveys, 415 from centers completed and returned
- Data based on telephone interviews and a focus group with child care providers

Source

Maine Child Care Market Rate and Workforce Study. 2002. Mills Consulting Group, funded by Office of Child Care and Head Start, Community Services Center, Department of Human Services, State of Maine, http://www.maine.gov/dhhs/ocfs/ec/occhs/workforcereport.pdf.

Minnesota

Child Care Workforce in Minnesota

- **Study Dates: 2006–2007**
- **Agency:** Minnesota Department of Human Services, Wilder Research

- The Minnesota Child Care Resource and Referral (CCR&R) Network provided Wilder Research a data file with all the current licensed family child care providers, child care centers, preschool sites and school-age care sites, including names, addresses, and phone numbers. The lists were stratified by metro area and greater Minnesota and then randomized.
- Surveys with 354 randomly selected licensed family child care providers and an over-sample of 149 American Indian, Hmong, Latino, and Somali licensed family child care providers; a two-part survey with 328 center-based programs and 1,162 directors and teaching staff; and nine focus groups with 77 providers and teachers
- Estimated 12,334 licensed family child care providers and center-based programs
- The estimated size of Minnesota's child care workforce is 36,500, which includes about 14,700 providers and paid assistants in the licensed home-based workforce and about 21,800 staff in the center-based workforce, including 2,050 directors, 9,150 teachers, 5,000 assistant teachers, and 5,600 aides

Source

Chase, R., C. Moore, S. Pierce, and J. Arnold. 2007. *Child care workforce in Minnesota, 2006 statewide study of demographics, training and professional development: Final report.* Minnesota Department of Human Services, http://www.wilder.org/download.0.html?report=1985.

New York

New York City Early Childhood Educators Survey

- **Study Date: 2006**
- **Agency:** NYC Early Childhood Professional Development Institute
- Surveyed directors, teachers, and assistant teachers in licensed community- and school-based early childhood centers in New York City serving children birth to 5 years old
- Including Head Start/Early Head Start, Universal Pre-kindergarten (UPK), Administration for Children Services (ACS), private, and blended/multitype
- A proportionate random sample of the centers was selected in such a way as to ensure sufficient representation from various types of community-based programs.
- **Sampling Population:** 2,727 licensed community and school based centers

- **Sample N:** 525 school-based UPK programs and 850 community-based centers within the 5 boroughs and 10 school districts

Source

Ochshorn, S., and M. Garcia. 2007. *Learning about the workforce: A profile of early childhood educators in New York City's community- and school-based centers.* New York City Early Childhood Professional Development Institute and Cornell University Early Childhood Program, http://www.earlychildhoodnyc.org/pdfs/eng/FinalReport.pdf.

North Carolina

North Carolina Child Care Workforce Survey

- **Study Dates: Spring and Summer 2003**
- **Agency:** Child Care Services Association and FPG Child Development Institute
- **Sample N:** Survey response rates were 78 percent of center directors (N = 2,203 director surveys collected), 52 percent of teachers (N = 13,120 teacher surveys collected), and 78 percent of family child care providers (N = 2,337 family child care provider surveys collected)
- Sampling based on county workforce size was used to create representative samples within each county.

Sources

Working in child care in Durham County: Durham Workforce Study 2009. Durham's Partnership for Children, a Smart Start Initiative, http://dpfc.net/Admin/uploads/photos/Documents/reports/WorkforceStudyFullReportFinal11.17.pdf.
Working in child care in North Carolina: The North Carolina Child Care Workforce Survey 2003. North Carolina Early Childhood Needs and Resources Assessment, Child Care Services Association, Frank Porter Graham Child Development Institute, http://www.childcareservices.org/_downloads/NC2003wfreport.pdf.

Ohio

Workforce Study of Ohio Early Childhood Centers

- **Study Date: April 2005**
- **Agency:** Ohio Child Care Resource and Referral Association
- Survey packets were sent to 3,600 randomly selected centers in April 2005, representing centers licensed by the Ohio Department of Job and Family Services (ODJFS) and, for the first time, programs licensed by the Ohio Department of Education (ODE)

- Overall, 989 centers responded, representing 388 ODE-licensed programs and 577 ODJFS-licensed programs. In the 2001 Ohio Association for the Education of Young Children (OAEYC) survey, 314 ODJFS-licensed centers responded.

Sources
2005 Workforce Study: Ohio early childhood centers, a profession divided. 2006. Columbus, OH: Ohio Child Care Resource and Referral Association.
2005 Workforce Study: Ohio early childhood centers, general analysis. 2006. Columbus, OH: Ohio Child Care Resource and Referral Association, http://www.ohpdnetwork.org/documents/workforce_general.pdf.

Oregon

- Few study/data details

Source
Investing in young kids = investing in their teachers: Building Oregon's early education workforce. 2008. Children's Institute, http://www.childinst.org/images/stories/ci_publications/ci-investing-in-youg-kids-2008.pdf.

Pennsylvania

Early Care and Education Provider Survey

- **Study Date: 2002**
- **Agency:** University of Pittsburgh Office of Child Development and Universities Children's Policy Collaborative (UCPC)
- **Sampling Population:** 15,220 early care and education sites, including 5,067 potential legally unregulated providers, representing a potentially exhaustive list of licensed and registered facilities within the classifications
- Attempted to contact 4,243 sites
- Interviews with 600 representative provider sites (stratified by six categories of providers and three categories of the population density of the county)

Source
Etheridge, W. A., R. B. McCall, C. J. Groark, K. E. Mehaffie, and R. Nelkin. 2002. *A baseline report of early care and education in Pennsylvania: The 2002 Early Care and Education Provider Survey*. University of Pittsburgh Office of Child Development and the Universities Children's Policy Collaborative (UCPC), http://www.prevention.psu.edu/ece/docs/FullReport1.pdf.

South Dakota

Child Care and Education Workforce Survey

- **Study Date: 2003**
- **General report not very detailed, not summarized in table**
- Early childhood workforce survey conducted by South Dakota KIDS COUNT and the University of South Dakota School of Education
- Survey mailed to child care centers, group family child care programs, Out-of-School-Time and Head Start programs in South Dakota
- Did not include Family Child Care Home programs
- 156 surveys returned (response rate of 40 percent)

    o 70 child care centers
    o 43 group family child care programs
    o 36 Out-of-School-Time programs
    o 7 Head Start programs

- Responding programs were located in 84 cities across the state, representing 46 counties.
- The results portray factors that influence approximately 1,900 program employees and 2,499 children.

Source

Who cares for children in South Dakota? Child Care and Early Education Workforce Survey executive summary. 2004. South Dakota KIDS COUNT and the University of South Dakota School of Education, http://dss.sd.gov/childcare/docs/whoc%20cares%20for%20 children%20in%20sd.pdf.

Utah

Study of the Childcare Workforce in Utah

- **Study Date: 2002**
- **Agency:** Mills Consulting Group, Inc. and Utah Office of Child Care
- A statewide survey of all licensed child care centers, school-age child care programs, and legally licensed exempt providers, and a sampling of residential certificate holders and licensed family and group providers

- **Sampling Population:** The survey sample was composed of all child care centers, school-age programs, and legally-licensed exempt programs.
- April 2002, a total of 1,415 surveys were sent to all child care centers, school-age programs, and legally licensed exempt programs, and to the sample of residential certificate holders and licensed family child care provider
- Two separate survey tools: one tailored for center-based, school-age and legally licensed exempt programs and another tailored for family child care providers and residential certificate holders
- **Sample N:** Response rates: 44 percent of child care programs (199 of 457), 62 percent of child care providers (594 of 958)

Source

A study of the child care workforce in Utah: Summary. 2002. Utah Office of Child Care, http://jobs.utah.gov/opencms/occ/occ2/learnmore/other/workforcesummary.pdf.

Vermont

Too small, not random

Defining Our Workforce Survey

- 2007
- 106 surveys collected, 91 at May conference, 11 through other sources

Vermont Afterschool Professionals Survey

- 2007
- 291 surveys

Source

Feal-Staub, L., and H. Morehouse. 2008. Afterschool professionals report for the National Career Pathways Project: Data collection, analysis, and synthesis, http://dcf.vermont.gov/sites/dcf/files/pdf/cdd/care/National_Career_Pathways_Project_Report.pdf.

Virginia

Child Care Workforce Study in Metro-Richmond, Virginia

- **Study Date: 2003**
- **Agency:** Voices for Virginia's Children
- There are approximately 350 child care centers in the metro-

Richmond region, providing early care and education to almost 11,000 children under the age of 6; there are an additional 332 family home providers in the metro-Richmond region, serving approximately 6,000 children.

- Surveys were mailed to child care centers to be completed by the directors and teachers and to family home providers.
- Between March 28, 2003, and July 15, 2003, 576 teacher surveys, 109 director surveys, and 121 family home provider surveys were completed and returned. The response rates were 17.4 percent (teacher surveys), 30.7 percent (director surveys), and 36.4 percent (family home provider surveys).
- Although the response rates may not have been as high as desired, the teachers, directors, and family home providers were evenly spread over the entire geographic area, and they came from a balanced sample of for-profit, non-profit, faith-based, licensed, and voluntarily registered sites.

Source

Child care workforce study in metro Richmond, Virginia: A status report on the child care workforce. 2004. Voices for Virginia's Children, http://www.vakids.org/pubs/Archives/ECE/workforce_study.pdf.

Wisconsin

Wisconsin Child Care Worker Survey

- **4 surveys: 1980, 1988, 1994, 2001**
- **Agency:** Wisconsin Early Childhood Association (WECA)
- 1980 (Edie and Frudden): 1,074 full-day child care centers and 278 family child care homes
- 1988 (Rily and Rodgers): 86 center directors, 171 teachers, 96 family day care providers
- 1994 (Burton et al.): stratified random sample of 104 center directors, 254 teachers, 185 licensed family care providers, 141 certified providers
- 2001 (Adams et al.): random sample of 2,000 child care programs; 342 center directors, 784 teachers, 452 family child care providers

Sources

Adams, D., M. Roach, D. Riley, and D. Edie. 2001. *Losing ground or keeping up? A report on the Wisconsin early care and education workforce.* Unpublished manuscript.

Adams, D., D. Durant, D. Edie, M. Ittig, D. Riley, M. Roach, S. Welsh, and D. Zeman. 2003. *Trends over time: Wisconsin's child care workforce.* Madison, WI: Wisconsin Early Childhood Association (WECA), http://wisconsinearlychildhood.org/.

Burton, A., M. Whitebook, L. Sakai, M. Babula, and P. Haack. 1994. *Valuable work, minimal rewards: A report on the Wisconsin child care work force.* National Center for the Early Childhood Work Force. Unpublished manuscript.

Edie, D., and G. Frudden. 1980. *A study of day care workers in Wisconsin.* Unpublished manuscript.

Riley, D., and K. Rodgers. 1988. *Pay, benefits, and job satisfaction of Wisconsin child care providers and early childhood teachers.* Unpublished manuscript.

VII. Single State; Cover Portion of B–5 Workforce and Settings, e.g., Prekindergarten

California

Changes in Child Care Staffing Study

- **Study Date: Three waves, 1994, 1996, 2000**
- **Agency:** Center for the Child Care Workforce (CCW)
- This study focuses on the staffing crisis in early childhood education and conducts a survey of caregivers in three areas of California.
- Based in three Bay Area communities of Santa Cruz, San Mateo, and Santa Clara in Northern California
- Longitudinal study of center caregivers from 1994 through 2000
- Data come from interviews and classroom observations
- **Sample Population:** NAEYC-accredited centers in three CA communities
- **Sample N 1994 and 1996:** 92 centers (observations and interviews in all), 2 preschool classrooms per center; 266 teaching staff observed in 1994; 260 staff observed in 1996

    o Generally classrooms serving 2.5- to 5-year-olds

- **Sample N 2000:** 75 centers (85 percent of 1996 sample), 43 observed, 32 interview only, observed 117 teaching staff, 83 teachers, 20 assistants, 14 teacher-directors; 75 directors—interviews providing information about staff at the center
- Total staff at 75 centers: 435 teachers, 182 assistants, 42 teacher-directors

Source
Whitebook, M., L. Sakai, E. Gerber, and C. Howes. 2001. *Then and now: Changes in child care staffing, 1994-2000.* Berkeley, CA: Center for the Study of Child Care Employment; San Francisco, CA: California Child Care Resource and Referral Network.

Massachusetts

Massachusetts Cost Quality Studies

- **Study Dates: 2000–2001**
- **Agency:** Wellesley Centers for Women and Abt Associates Inc.
- Studies in three parts: Center Study, Public Preschool Study, and Family Child Care Study
- Focuses on those serving 3–5-year-olds
- 2004: centers with capacity to serve 91,232 3–5-year-olds, 7,369 family child care homes with capacity for 29,476; Head Start providing preschool education for 12,969 children in 163 programs; 22,533 children ages 3–5 enrolled in preschool classrooms in 466 public schools

Source

Marshall, N., J. Dennehy, C. Johnson-Staub, and W. Robeson. 2005. *Massachusetts capacity study research brief: Characteristics of the current early education and care workforce serving 3–5-year-olds.* Wellesley Centers for Women and Abt Associates Inc., http://www.wcwonline.org/earlycare/workforcefindings2005.pdf.

Cost Quality (CQ) Center Study

- **Study Date: 2000**
- **Agency:** Wellesley Centers for Women and Abt Associates Inc.
- Random sample of 90 community-based centers serving preschoolers on a full-day, full-year basis; 65 percent response rate
- Drawn from across the state in proportion to the region's market share of the state's center-based ECE market

Source

Marshall, N. L., C. L. Creps, N. R. Burstein, F. B. Glantz, W. Wagner Robeson, and S. Barnett. 2001. *The cost and quality of full-day, year-round early care and education in Massachusetts: Preschool classrooms.* Wellesley, MA: Wellesley Centers for Women and Abt Associates Inc.

CQ Public Preschool Study

- **Study Date: 2000**
- **Agency:** Wellesley Centers for Women and Abt Associates Inc.
- Random sample of 95 school-based, publicly administered preschool classrooms, from a list of all schools housing preschool classrooms, as reported to the Department of Education by school districts from around the state

Source

Marshall, N. L., C. L. Creps, N. R. Burstein, F. B. Glantz, W. Wagner Robeson, S. Barnett, J. Schimmenti, and N. Keefe. 2002. *Early care and education in Massachusetts public school preschool classrooms.* Wellesley, MA: Wellesley Centers for Women and Abt Associates Inc.

CQ Family Child Care Study

- **Study Dates: 2000–2001**
- **Agency:** Wellesley Centers for Women and Abt Associates Inc.
- Random sample of licensed family child care homes (FCCHs) from MA Office for Child Care Services (OCCS)
- 203 participating in study (57 percent of those selected)

Source

Marshall, N. L., C. L. Creps, N. R. Burstein, K. E. Cahill, W. Wagner Robeson, S. Y. Wang, N. Keefe, J. Schimmenti, F. B. Glantz. 2005. *Massachusetts family child care Today: A report of the findings of the Massachusetts Cost/Quality Study: Family child care homes.* Wellesley, MA: Wellesley Centers for Women and Abt Associates Inc.

FEDERAL DATA SOURCES FOR UNDERSTANDING THE EARLY CHILDHOOD CARE AND EDUCATION WORKFORCE: A BACKGROUND PAPER
April 22, 2011

Prepared by Dixie Sommers, Assistant Commissioner, Bureau of Labor Statistics, for the Institute of Medicine–National Research Council's Early Childhood Care and Education Workforce: Phase One Planning Committee

PURPOSE

This background paper provides information about data sources produced by the Bureau of Labor Statistics (BLS) and the Census Bureau relevant to understanding the Early Childhood Care and Education (ECCE) workforce. The information presented is based on discussions of the workshop planning committee.

The paper begins with descriptions of the two major classification systems used in BLS and Census data, the North American Industry Classification System (NAICS) and the Standard Occupational Classification (SOC). Both the occupational and industry dimensions of the workforce are useful in identifying ECCE jobs, workers, and establishments and understanding their characteristics and trends. In general, industry classifications depict the economy according to the type of products or services produced, while occupations are based on the type of work performed. Understanding the foundations of the classifications and how they are developed and revised will assist ECCE researchers both in their use of industry and occupational data and in preparing recommendations for the next NAICS and SOC revisions.

The descriptions of the NAICS and SOC are followed by a discussion of issues these classifications present for ECCE workforce analysis. Additional issues concerning BLS and Census data (referred to as the "standard data sources") for ECCE purposes are also discussed.

The remainder of the paper profiles the relevant data sources from the Department of Labor and the Census Bureau, using a template format to present key metadata, and including a brief assessment of advantages and limitations of the data sources for ECCE purposes.

NORTH AMERICAN INDUSTRY CLASSIFICATION SYSTEM

Federal economic data often provide information about industries, such as manufacturing or retail trade. In federal statistics, the Office of

Management and Budget (OMB) requires that industries be classified using the North American Industry Classification System or NAICS.

NAICS groups establishments into industries based on the similarity of their production processes. An establishment, as defined by the BLS, is a physical location of a certain economic activity—for example, a factory, mine, store, or office. An enterprise[10] (a private firm, government, or non-profit organization) can consist of a single establishment or multiple establishments. Depending on their products or activities, all establishments in an enterprise may be classified in one industry, or they may be classified in different industries. In the ECCE context, establishments include child care centers, schools, private homes, and any other type of establishment where ECCE services are provided.

The 2007 NAICS is a tiered system with five levels, ranging from 20 industry sectors to 1,175 detailed industries. Each establishment is classified into only one of the detailed industries based on its principal product or activity, usually determined by annual sales volume. Each detailed industry has a code, title, and definition; it may also have illustrative examples of products or services and cross-references to other industries. The coding system uses a six-digit code, with the first two digits indicating the major industry sector.

Developing and Revising the NAICS

The NAICS replaced the Standard Industry Classification, or SIC, in 1997, providing a common industry classification for use in the United States, Canada, and Mexico. The NAICS structure was developed through trilateral meetings to consider public proposals from each country. In the United States, OMB established the interagency Economic Classification Policy Committee (ECPC), chaired by the Census Bureau, to develop classification proposals.[11]

NAICS is developed to serve statistical purposes, such as collecting and tabulating statistical information; while it may be used for administrative, regulatory or taxation purposes, these purposes played no role in its development or revision.

The most recent edition is the 2007 NAICS.[12] The ECPC has provided

---

[10] "Enterprise" in this context is used differently from "enterprise" as defined in the conceptual definition presented at the workshop.

[11] Information about the NAICS is available at http://www.census.gov/eos/www/naics/. Information about BLS application of the NAICS is available at http://www.bls.gov/bls/naics.htm.

[12] In both the NAICS and SOC, the edition year is not the year of publication but the year in which implementation is expected, ideally the reference year of the first data on the new classification.

recommendations to OMB for the 2012 revision, and OMB is expected to publish the final 2012 NAICS soon. In preparing the 2012 revision, OMB and the ECPC solicited public input through three *Federal Register* Notices. The NAICS is revised on a 5-year cycle, with the next revision scheduled for implementation in 2017.

Standard Occupational Classification

Labor market data often provide information about occupations: the number of workers, trends in employment, pay and benefits, demographic characteristics, and other items. To ensure that occupational data from across the federal statistical system are comparable and can be used together in analysis, OMB has established the Standard Occupational Classification, or SOC.[13]

The 2010 SOC is a tiered system with four levels, ranging from 23 major groups to 840 detailed occupations. Each worker is classified into only one of the detailed occupations based on the tasks he or she performs. Each detailed occupation has a code, title, definition, and may have illustrative examples. The coding system uses a six-digit code, with the first two digits indicating the major occupation group. An online "direct match title file" provides job titles that should be assigned to one and only one detailed SOC occupation.

Developing and Revising the SOC The SOC was first issued in 1977, with a subsequent revision in 1980, but neither of these versions was widely used. With the implementation of the 2000 SOC, for the first time all major occupational data sources produced by the federal statistical system provided comparable data, greatly improving the usefulness of the data. The most recent revision resulted in the 2010 SOC, which is now being implemented in federal data collection programs.

As with the NAICS, the SOC is developed to serve statistical purposes. While the SOC may be used for other purposes, these purposes play no role in its development or revision.

Revising the SOC is a multiyear process, as demonstrated by the milestones for the 2010 revision. The process began in 2005, when OMB convened the interagency Standard Occupational Classification Policy Committee (SOCPC), chaired by the Bureau of Labor Statistics. The SOCPC is charged with developing recommendations to OMB for changes in the SOC. After receiving public comments in response to two *Federal Register* Notices, issued in May 2006 and May 2008, the SOCPC made final recom-

---

[13] Much of this discussion of the SOC is drawn from the Introduction to the *2010 Standard Occupational Classification Manual*. See http://www.bls.gov/soc/#publications.

mendations to OMB that were published in January 2009. The 2010 SOC Manual, which provided the definitions, was published in March 2009.

The SOCPC has proposed that the next revision of the SOC will result in a 2018 edition, with the revision work expected to begin in 2013. This revision schedule is intended to minimize disruption to data providers, producers, and users by promoting simultaneous adoption of revised occupational and industry classification systems for those data series that use both. This is best accomplished by timing revisions of the SOC for the years following NAICS revisions. The next such year is 2018, which has the additional benefit of coinciding with the beginning year of the American Community Survey's next 5-year set of surveys. OMB intends to consider revisions of the SOC for 2018 and every 10 years thereafter.

SOC Classification Principles The Classification Principles listed in Box B-1 are the basis of SOC structure. The SOCPC referred to these principles in making decisions about the creation or modification of detailed occupations and their placement in the SOC. Thus, in considering any recommendation for changing or adding an occupation, the SOCPC needs information about how the recommendation is consistent with the Classification Principles.

Classification Principles 1 and 2 are fundamental to the SOC and apply across all occupations. Because the purpose of the SOC is for preparing statistical information on the workforce, it is important to specify its scope. Principle 1 does this by specifying that the SOC covers all work performed for pay or profit, and specifying that occupations unique to volunteer work are not included. In the ECCE context, the SOC is used to classify workers who provide early childhood care and instruction and who receive wage or salary pay or self-employment income for providing these services. Specific SOC occupations related to these activities are discussed later in this paper.

Classification Principle 2 establishes the work performed as the main criterion for establishing a detailed occupation and determining where to place it in the structure. Thus, the SOCPC needs information describing the tasks performed by workers in an occupation. The SOCPC uses this information to evaluate whether the tasks performed in a new occupation recommended for inclusion are sufficiently different from tasks performed in existing occupations, and to determine where in the classification structure an occupation should be placed. In revising existing occupations, the SOCPC considers whether tasks have changed since the last revision. As noted in Principle 2, skills, education, or training are sometimes used to guide the classification decisions.

Classification Principle 3 is critical for classification of managers,

**BOX B-1
2010 SOC Classification Principles**

1. The SOC covers all occupations in which work is performed for pay or profit, including work performed in family-operated enterprises by family members who are not directly compensated. It excludes occupations unique to volunteers. Each occupation is assigned to only one occupational category at the lowest level of the classification.

2. Occupations are classified based on work performed and, in some cases, on the skills, education, and/or training needed to perform the work at a competent level.

3. Workers primarily engaged in planning and directing are classified in management occupations in Major Group 11-0000. Duties of these workers may include supervision.

4. Supervisors of workers in Major Groups 13-0000 through 29-0000 usually have work experience and perform activities similar to those of the workers they supervise, and therefore are classified with the workers they supervise.

5. Workers in Major Group 31-0000 Health Care Support Occupations assist and are usually supervised by workers in Major Group 29-0000 Health Care Practitioners and Technical Occupations. Therefore, there are no first-line supervisor occupations in Major Group 31-0000.

6. Workers in Major Groups 33-0000 through 53-0000 whose primary duty is supervising are classified in the appropriate first-line supervisor category because their work activities are distinct from those of the workers they supervise.

7. Apprentices and trainees are classified with the occupations for which they are being trained, while helpers and aides are classified separately because they are not in training for the occupation they are helping.

8. If an occupation is not included as a distinct detailed occupation in the structure, it is classified in an appropriate "All Other," or residual, occupation. "All Other" occupations are placed in the structure when it is determined that the detailed occupations comprising a broad occupation group do not account for all of the workers in the group. These occupations appear as the last occupation in the group with a code ending in "9" and are identified in their title by having "All Other" appear at the end.

9. The U.S. Bureau of Labor Statistics and the U.S. Census Bureau are charged with collecting and reporting data on total U.S. employment across the full spectrum of SOC major groups. Thus, for a detailed occupation to be included in the SOC, either the Bureau of Labor Statistics or the Census Bureau must be able to collect and report data on that occupation.

SOURCE: Standard Occupational Classification Manual 2010, Office of Management and Budget.

focusing on duties of "planning and directing." The principle recognizes that managers may also supervise other workers. In the setting of a small child care center, for example, the center director would be classified as a manager, not a supervisor, although this individual may supervise some or all of the other workers in the center.

Classification Principle 4 indicates how supervisors of workers in classified in Major Occupation Groups 13 through 29 are classified. In these Major Groups, there are no specific supervisory occupations. Instead, supervisors who also perform work similar to that of the workers they supervise are classified with those workers. In the ECCE context, this principle is relevant for teaching occupations, found in Major Group 25. For example, a lead teacher who teaches preschool but also supervises other preschool teachers would be classified in one of the two preschool teaching occupations: 25-2011 Preschool Teachers, Except Special Education, or 25-5051 Special Education Teachers, Preschool.

Classification of supervisors of teachers is different from how supervisors of child care workers are classified. Child care workers are in Major Group 39, where Classification Principle 6 applies and specific supervisory occupations are included in the SOC. The supervisory detailed occupation relevant to ECCE is 39-1021 First-line Supervisors of Personal Care Workers.

Classification Principle 7 concerns the classification of apprentices. While the principle mentions helpers and aides, these are generally not child care helpers or aides. This principle is used, for example, to classify workers who perform tasks similar to those of a construction helper but who are in a carpenter apprentice program and are helping carpenters as part of the apprenticeship training. These workers would be classified as in the occupation for which they are being trained, i.e., carpenter.

SOC Coding Guidelines In addition to the Classification Principles, the SOCPC developed the Coding Guidelines show in Box B-2 to assist users in consistently assigning SOC codes and titles to survey responses and in other coding activities. The Coding Guidelines reflect the reality of many workplaces—that individual workers may perform a variety of tasks that could be classified into more than one occupation. The guidelines help produced consistent treatment of these situations.

Coding Guideline 2 is important in understanding how workers who perform a range of duties are classified, probably a common situation in smaller ECCE establishments. Except for teachers, the main criterion is the skill level required by the various tasks. For example, a child care center director who also teaches would be classified as 11-9031 Education Administrators, Preschool and Childcare Center/Program, if the directing tasks are regarded as requiring higher skills than the teaching tasks. If the

---

BOX B-2
2010 SOC Coding Guidelines

1. A worker should be assigned to an SOC occupation code based on work performed.

2. When workers in a single job could be coded in more than one occupation, they should be coded in the occupation that requires the highest level of skill. If there is no measurable difference in skill requirements, workers should be coded in the occupation in which they spend the most time. Workers whose job is to teach at different levels (e.g., elementary, middle, or secondary) should be coded in the occupation corresponding to the highest educational level they teach.

3. Data collection and reporting agencies should assign workers to the most detailed occupation possible. Different agencies may use different levels of aggregation, depending on their ability to collect data.

4. Workers who perform activities not described in any distinct detailed occupation in the SOC structure should be coded in an appropriate "All Other" or residual occupation. These residual occupational categories appear as the last occupation in a group with a code ending in "9" and are identified by having the words "All Other" appear at the end of the title.

5. Workers in Major Groups 33-0000 through 53-0000 who *spend 80 percent or more of their time performing supervisory activities* are coded in the appropriate first-line supervisor category in the SOC. In these same Major Groups (33-0000 through 53-0000), persons with supervisory duties who *spend less than 80 percent of their time supervising* are coded with the workers they supervise.

6. Licensed and non-licensed workers performing the same work should be coded together in the same detailed occupation, except where specified otherwise in the SOC definition.

SOURCE: Standard Occupational Classification Manual 2010, Office of Management and Budget.

---

skill levels are regarded as similar, time spent directing versus teaching should be used as a tie-breaker.

Teachers who teach at more than one level should be classified at the higher level. For example a teacher working at both the preschool and elementary levels should be classified in an elementary school teacher occupation.

Coding Guideline 5 deals with classification of supervisors who also perform non-supervisory work. For example, a worker who supervises child care workers may also perform child care tasks. Whether this worker is classified with 39-1021 First-line Supervisors of Personal Care Workers or with 39-9011 Childcare Workers should depend on the amount of time spent supervising versus providing care.

Using the NAICS and SOC to Understand the ECCE Workforce

Discussions with members of the workshop planning committee identified a number of difficulties in using data based on the NAICS and SOC to understand the ECCE workforce. The following issues are detailed here:

1. *The 2010 SOC does not consistently distinguish workers who care for or instruct children from birth through age five (the B–5 population) from those who care for or instruct school-aged children.*
2. *The SOC distinction between child care worker and preschool teacher does not reflect the work performed.*
3. *The relevant NAICS industries do not identify child care or instructional services by age of the children served.*
4. *Industry data classified by NAICS cannot be used to identify preschool or child care services provided by establishments whose primary activity is not child day care services.*

1. *The 2010 SOC does not consistently distinguish workers who care for or instruct children from birth through age five (the B–5 population) from those who care for or instruct school-aged children.*

ECCE researchers indicate that the duties and responsibilities involved in caring for or instructing younger children are different from those required for school-aged children. Programs for school-aged children may range from centers to school-based programs, and include recreational and after-school instruction programs. These activities may be staffed with workers classified in various SOC occupations, including teachers, child care workers, recreation workers, and others.

The 2010 SOC includes the occupations where workers who provide care or instruction to the B–5 population are classified, as well as relevant education administrators and the supervisors of child care workers. (See Table B-21.) Only two occupations listed specifically identify and are limited to the B–5 population: 25-2011 Preschool Teachers, Except Special Education, and 25-2051 Special Education Teachers, Preschool.

SOC 11-9031 Education Administrators, Preschool and Child Care Center/Program, likely serve mostly the B–5 population. However, "Child Care Center/Program" could include centers or programs serving mainly older children. The extent to which this is the case is not known from the standard data sources.

In all the remaining occupations listed, the occupational classification alone does not distinguish workers who serve only or primarily the B–5 population.

2. *The SOC distinction between child care worker and preschool teacher does not reflect the work performed.*

The SOC distinguishes 25-2011 Preschool Teachers, Except Special Education from 39-9011 Child Care Workers based on the work activities performed, which are described in the occupational definitions in Table B-21. Generally, the distinction is that Preschool Teachers provide instruction while Child Care Workers perform tasks other than instruction.

ECCE researchers indicate that this distinction does not reflect practices and standards in the field. For example, the National Association for the Education of Young Children (NAEYC) conducts a voluntary accreditation system that sets professional standards for early childhood education programs and accredits programs that prepare early childhood educators.[14] NAEYC also has developed standards for "Developmentally Appropriate Practice" in early childhood programs that include practices and standards related to encouraging cognitive, social, and other development of young children.[15] Similarly, the National Board for Professional Teaching Standards has developed standards for teaching children age 3 through 8, and conducts a teacher certification program.[16]

The Employment and Training Administration's Occupational Information Network or O*NET program gathers information on tasks, skills, and many other data items from incumbent workers in specific SOC occupations. Of interest here is that the task list for Child Care Workers includes tasks that may be considered beyond custodial care activities. Examples include "Create developmentally appropriate lesson plans," "Support children's emotional and social development, encouraging understanding of others and positive self-concepts" and "Identify signs of emotional or developmental problems in children and bring them to parents' or guardians' attention."[17]

3. *The relevant NAICS industries do not identify child care or instructional services by age of the children served.*

For each of the four components of ECCE, the relevant 2007 NAICS industries and their definitions are listed in Table B-22. The identification of specific NAICS for the first three components—school-based, center-based, and formal Family Child Care (FCC) home-based services—are rel-

---

[14] See http://www.naeyc.org/positionstatements/dap.
[15] See http://www.naeyc.org/positionstatements/dap.
[16] See http://www.nbpts.org/.
[17] O*NET Online, http://www.onetonline.org/.

TABLE B-21 2010 SOC Detailed Occupations Most Relevant to ECCE

Code and Title	Definition	Direct Match Titles*
11-9031 Education Administrators, Preschool and Childcare Center/Program	Plan, direct, or coordinate the academic and nonacademic activities of preschool and child care centers or programs. Exclude "Preschool Teachers" (25-2011).	• Child care center administrator • Child care center director • Early Head Start director • Head Start director • Prekindergarten program coordinator • Preschool director
25-2011 Preschool Teachers, Except Special Education	Instruct preschool-aged children in activities designed to promote social, physical, and intellectual growth needed for primary school in preschool, day care center, or other child development facility. Substitute teachers are included in "Teachers and Instructors, All Other" (25-3099). May be required to hold state certification. Excludes "Child Care Workers" (39-9011) and "Special Education Teachers" (25-2050).	• Early childhood teacher • Head Start teacher • Nursery school teacher • Nursery teacher • Prekindergarten teacher • Preschool teacher
25-2051 Special Education Teachers, Preschool	Teach preschool school subjects to educationally and physically handicapped students. Includes teachers who specialize and work with audibly and visually handicapped students and those who teach basic academic and life processes skills to the mentally impaired. Substitute teachers are included in "Teachers and Instructors, All Other" (25-3099).	• Early childhood special education teacher • Early childhood special educator • Prekindergarten special education teacher
25-9041 Teacher Assistants	Perform duties that are instructional in nature or deliver direct services to students or parents. Serve in a position for which a teacher has ultimate responsibility for the design and implementation of educational programs and services. Excludes "Graduate Teaching Assistants" (25-1191).	• Basic skills improvement program instructional aide • Classroom aide • Educational assistant teacher • Gifted and talented student education aide • Instructional aide • Instructional assistant

		• Learning support aide • Paraeducator • Public health training assistant • Reading aide • Special education aide • Special education classroom aide • Special education instructional assistant • Special education paraeducator • Special education paraprofessional • Special education teaching assistant • Teacher aide
39-1021 First-Line Supervisors of Personal Service Workers	Directly supervise and coordinate activities of personal service workers, such as flight attendants, hairdressers, or caddies.	• Animal trainer supervisor • Caddy master • Head butler • Recreation attendant supervisor
39-9011 Child Care Workers	Attend to children at schools, businesses, private households, and child care institutions. Perform a variety of tasks, such as dressing, feeding, bathing, and overseeing play. Excludes "Preschool Teachers, Except Special Education" (25-2011) and "Teacher Assistants" (25-9041).	• Au pair • Baby sitter • Before and after school day care worker • Child care aide • Child care attendant • Child care worker • Day care attendant • Day care worker • Day care aide • Day care provider • Governess • Nanny • Nursery day care worker • Playground aide

NOTE: ECCE: Early Childhood Care Education; SOC: Standard Occupational Classification; SOCPC: Standard Occupational Classification Policy Committee.
* Direct match titles are titles that the SOCPC has agreed match only one SOC occupation. These may not be the only job titles relevant to the detailed occupation, however.

TABLE B-22 2007 NAICS Detailed Industries Most Relevant to ECCE Components

ECCE Component	NAICS Code and Title	NAICS Definition	NAICS Illustrative Examples
School-based	611110 Elementary and secondary schools	This industry comprises establishments primarily engaged in furnishing academic courses and associated course work that comprise a basic preparatory education. A basic preparatory education ordinarily constitutes kindergarten through 12th grade. This industry includes school boards and school districts.	• Elementary schools • Parochial schools, elementary • High schools • Primary schools • Kindergartens • Schools for the physically disabled, elementary or secondary • Military academies, elementary or secondary
Center-based Formal family child care (FCC) home-based services Family, friend, and neighbor (FFN): self-employed, providing care in own home.	624410 Child day care services	This industry comprises establishments primarily engaged in providing day care of infants or children. These establishments generally care for preschool children, but may care for older children when they are not in school and may also offer prekindergarten educational programs.	• Child day care babysitting services • Nursery schools • Child or infant day care centers • Preschool centers
Family, friend, and neighbor (FFN): Workers receiving a wage from the householder (usually the parent) and providing care in the child's home.	814110 Private households	This industry comprises private households primarily engaged in employing workers on or about the premises in activities primarily concerned with the operation of the household. These private households may employ individuals, such as cooks, maids, nannies, butlers, and outside workers, such as gardeners, caretakers, and other maintenance workers.	None

NOTE: ECCE: Early Childhood Care Education; NAICS: North American Industry Classification System.

atively straightforward. The industry classification of the Family, Friend, and Neighbor (FFN) component is more complex, however.

The FFN component includes paid services provided in the caregiver's home, with the payment from the parents or from a third party, such as a voucher program. Generally, these caregivers would be considered self-employed. FFN caregivers who are providing paid services in the child's home, and who are paid by the householder (most likely the child's parent) would be classified as working in the Private Households industry. In both instances, accurate measurement depends on these workers' responses to the household survey questions discussed later in this paper.

As to the issue of services according to the age of the children served, only the description for NAICS 624410 Child Day Care Services references preschool age children, which is likely the dominant population served by establishments classified here. The illustrative examples for this industry, shown in Table B-22, suggest this may be the case: Child day care babysitting services, Nursery schools, Child or infant day care centers, and Preschool centers. However, the standard labor force and employment data sources provide no information on the actual mix of B–5 and older children served. The extent of the limitation of this NAICS code for ECCE purposes is not known but may be small.

4. *Industry data classified by NAICS cannot be used to identify preschool or child care services provided by establishments whose primary activity is not child day care services.*

Establishments are classified in the NAICS according to their primary activity. Thus, only establishments that provide child care services as their primary activity will be classified in NAICS 624410 Child Day Care Services. Child care centers are operated by establishments in other industries, and the number of such centers and their employment cannot be identified using standard industry data sources classified by the NAICS.

An important example is school-based ECCE programs operated by elementary and secondary schools. Preschools and child care centers are located in schools whose primary activities are providing elementary and secondary education and are classified in NAICS 611110, Elementary and Secondary Schools. Not all schools have ECCE programs, however. Thus, the NAICS designation alone is not sufficient to identify establishments providing ECCE services. Additional information about schools is needed.

Other Federal Data Issues for ECCE

In addition to issues related to the classifications, several measurement issues have been identified in using BLS and Census data sources for ECCE workforce analysis. The following issues are discussed here:

5. *Where the 2010 SOC does distinguish workers who provide care or instruction to the B–5 population, the distinction is not available in data collected through household surveys.*
6. *The standard data sources provide little information on the type of preparation by early childhood care and education workers.*
7. *It is difficult to identify formal Family Child Care home-based care services and informal Family, Friend, and Neighbor care services in the standard data sources.*
8. *The Current Population Survey does not provide statistically reliable data for small domains because of the limited sample size.*

5. *Where the 2010 SOC does distinguish workers who provide care or instruction to the B–5 population, the distinction is not available in data collected through household surveys.*

In general, household surveys provide less occupational and industry detail than establishment surveys, because there is less information available for assigning classification codes. An important example of this limitation is SOC 25-2011 Preschool Teachers, Except Special Education. The Current Population Survey (CPS) and the American Community Survey (ACS) provide data for SOC 25-2010 Preschool and Kindergarten Teachers, but not separately for preschool versus kindergarten teachers. Similar groupings of SOC occupations are made for education administrators and special education teachers, where no distinctions as to the level of education are indicated.

Because the CPS and ACS are the main sources of demographic information of workers by occupation, this limitation results in lack of data on educational attainment, gender, age, race/ethnicity, and other characteristics of workers in the occupations of interest to ECCE, and that facilitates comparison with other occupations. In addition, the CPS and ACS are the source of employment data by occupation for workers in private households.

The BLS Occupational Employment Statistics (OES) survey does produce data specifically for Education Administrators, Preschool and Child Care Center/Program and for Preschool Teachers, Except Special Education. With implementation of the 2010 SOC, BLS will also begin publishing data for 25-2051 Special Education Teachers, Preschool; these new data will be available starting in the spring of 2012. The OES survey provides data on employment levels and wages, total and by industry and by geographic area; it does not provide demographic information, however, nor does it include private households.

6. *The standard data sources provide little information on the type of preparation by early childhood care and education workers.*

Some members of the workshop planning committee identified the need for information about the preparation of ECCE workers, such as general educational attainment, early childhood-specific education, professional development and training, and work experience. The standard household surveys (CPS and ACS) provide only data on formal educational attainment by occupation. The usefulness of this information is limited by the Census groupings of SOC occupations, as described in item 5 above.

The ACS recently began publishing data on bachelor's degree field of study. These data can be tabulated by occupation and other characteristics. Field of degree data are used by the National Science Foundation to study the characteristics of the population with science and engineering degrees and occupations. The categories reported in the data are rather broad, but do include Education as a specific category.[18]

None of the standard labor force and employment surveys contain questions on more detailed preparation, such as types of courses taken, more specific information on field of study, or credentials obtained other than formal educational attainment. Other data sources must be used to obtain this type of data.

7. *It is difficult to identify formal Family Child Care home-based care services and informal Family, Friend, and Neighbor care services in the standard data sources.*

This issue poses different measurement problems for establishment versus household data, which are discussed separately below. In general, however, there are two difficulties: (1) whether and how formal FCC home-based services are captured in statistical sources and (2) the use of different concepts by ECCE researchers and statistical agencies regarding FFN care.

In the FCC case, care is provided for pay in a formal setting that is located at the caregiver's home. The key distinction is the "formal setting," that is, a home-based child care business, usually operated by a

---

[18] See /www.census.gov/acs/www/Downloads/data_documentation/SubjectDefinitions/ 2009_ACSSubjectDefinitions.pdf.

sole proprietor. The FCC concept is compatible with statistical concepts of establishment (the home-based business is the establishment) and the economic relationship between the FCC proprietor and the customer, who pays the proprietor directly or creates an arrangement for payment through a third party, such as voucher program. In practice, however, the standard establishment and household surveys do not distinguish home-based formal settings from other formal settings, such as center-based care.

The FFN concept is based on personal relationships between the caregiver, on the one hand, and the child and parent, on the other. The caregiver is a family member, friend, or neighbor of the child or parent, and is providing care on an informal paid basis, either in the caregiver's home or the child's home. In contrast, labor force concepts turn on the employment relationship, that is, whether a worker is paid through a wage or salary or earns income through self-employment, and the location of the activity. Measurement depends on either the coverage of the paid activity by the Unemployment Insurance (UI) system or on the way individuals respond to questions on household surveys. Neither establishment nor household surveys take personal or family relationships into account in employment concepts or measurement (except for "unpaid family workers" in household surveys).

Establishment Data Four components of the ECCE service delivery system are: center-based, school-based, formal FCC home-based services, and FFN services. Center-based and school-based programs are generally straightforward in where they are classified in the NAICS, as seen in Table B-22, and therefore in their inclusion in the BLS establishment list. The BLS establishment list is derived from the employer's quarterly state UI payroll tax reports. Thus, whether the activity is covered by state UI laws determines whether the establishment is identified, coded, and included in the BLS universe for its establishment surveys. The UI tax reports provide data on the establishment's total employment and payroll for workers covered by the UI system, and are coded by NAICS, geographic location, ownership (public or private), and a variety of other characteristics.

Formal FCC home-based services and informal FFN services are more complicated. Generally these complications turn on two questions: (1) whether the activity is covered by the state UI law, and (2) how proprietors of FCC home-based services are counted.

UI coverage of formal FCC home-based services and FFN services is depicted in Table B-23. This is a general view, as specific coverage varies somewhat from state to state. As noted in the chart, UI coverage is subject to meeting a threshold amount of wages paid in a recent period, and

TABLE B-23 Unemployment Insurance Coverage for FCC and FFN Child Care Services Workers

Employment Relationship	Formal Family Child Care (FCC) Home-Based Care	Family, Friend, or Neighbor (FFN) Care
Proprietors		
Incorporated	Covered	Not applicable
Not incorporated	Not covered, considered self-employed	Not applicable
Paid employees of proprietor		
Incorporated	Covered	Not applicable
Not incorporated	Covered	Not applicable
Paid employees of householders	Not applicable	May be covered as "domestic service"
Self-employed non-proprietors	Not applicable	Not covered

NOTE: UI coverage is subject to meeting the required amount of wages paid during a recent quarter or year, which varies by state. Wage requirements for "domestic service" are usually different than those for other types of workers. See http://www.ows.doleta.gov/unemploy/pdf/uilawcompar/2010/coverage.pdf.

requirements usually differ for "domestic service," that is, employees paid by a householder.[19]

For FCC proprietors, whether they are UI-covered and therefore counted in the establishment's reported employment depends on whether the home-based business is incorporated. Officers of incorporated businesses—in this case, proprietors of incorporated home-based businesses—are generally considered paid employees.[20] These establishments would be classified according to the services provided, probably in NAICS 624410 Child Day Care Services, and would be in the universe for BLS establishment surveys. Proprietors are relevant only for FCC and not for FFN care. Paid employees of FCC proprietors are covered by UI, regardless of whether the business is incorporated.

The only instance where workers providing FFN services are covered by UI is where a householder pays the caregiver as an employee and

---

[19] "Domestic service" is defined in Federal Unemployment Tax Act (FUTA) regulations to include babysitting. See http://edocket.access.gpo.gov/cfr_2010/aprqtr/pdf/26cfr31.3306(c)(2)-1.pdf. All state UI laws cover domestic service, although the specific provisions are different from the federal coverage in a few states.

[20] For FUTA purposes, corporate officers are considered paid employees. Some states have enacted exclusions from state UI coverage. See page 11 of http://www.ows.doleta.gov/unemploy/pdf/uilawcompar/2010/coverage.pdf.

the wages paid meet the threshold level. The paid employee may be a family member, friend, or neighbor, but also could be a nanny, who is not included in the FFN concept. The household would be considered to be the establishment, and would be classified in NAICS 814110 Private Households. These establishments are on the BLS establishment list, but no BLS establishment survey includes this industry.

Household Data The CPS and ACS ask questions about the respondent's employment status, occupation, industry, and class of worker status (wage and salary, unincorporated self-employed, and unpaid family workers). The classification of individual workers depends on how they respond to these questions and the amount of detail they provide. Table B-24 presents the relevant ACS questions[21] and should be helpful in understanding how proprietors are counted in household data. Similar or identical questions are used on the CPS.

Proprietors of home-based FCC services may answer question 41 as either self-employed in an incorporated business or self-employed in an unincorporated business and will be classified as either wage and salary workers (if incorporated) or self-employed workers (if not incorporated). Employees working for the FCC proprietor would probably respond as employees of private for-profit business or individual, and would be classified as wage and salary workers.[22] The Current Population Survey question similar to question 41, the first response item does not include working as an employee of an individual.

To code the industry and occupation responses, the Census Bureau maintains industry and occupation title indexes.[23] For the industry questions, responses such as "child care" and "day care" are coded to the Census industry equivalent of NAICS 624410 Child Day Care Services. Census coding procedures may use occupational responses to aid in coding the industry. For example, responses indicating self-employed with the occupation babysitter, and working in the home of others, are coded to the Census industry equivalent of NAICS 814110 Private Households.

---

[21] See http://www.census.gov/acs/www/Downloads/questionnaires/2011/Quest11.pdf.

[22] CPS interviewer instructions include the following for child care workers: "Child care including foster parents WHERE a person works is important in determining the correct class of worker for child care workers. Persons who care for children in the child's (that is the parent's) home are private for profit employees. This includes a babysitter for an evening or a person regularly working during the day. One of the private categories is also correct for those who work in day care centers and other non-government institutional settings. The institution may be either for profit or not for profit. A person who cares for children in the caregiver's home is self employed. This includes foster parents who receive a fee for caring for children." http://www.census.gov/apsd/techdoc/cps/CPS_Interviewing_Manual_July2008rv.pdf, page C4-33.

[23] See http://www.census.gov/hhes/www/ioindex/ioindex.html.

TABLE B-24 American Community Survey Questions on Class of Worker, Industry, and Occupation

Question	Question	Responses Coded to
41	Was this person–*Mark (X) ONE box.* ☐ an employee of a PRIVATE FOR-PROFIT company or business, or of an individual, for wages, salary, or commissions? ☐ an employee of a PRIVATE NOT-FOR-PROFIT, tax-exempt, or charitable organization? ☐ a local GOVERNMENT employee (city, county, etc.)? ☐ a state GOVERNMENT employee? ☐ a federal GOVERNMENT employee? ☐ SELF-EMPLOYED in own NOT INCORPORATED business, professional practice, or farm? ☐ SELF-EMPLOYED in own INCORPORATED business, professional practice, or farm? ☐ working WITHOUT PAY in family business or farm?	Class of worker: • Wage and salary • Unincorporated self-employed • Unpaid family workers Ownership: • Federal • State • Local • Private
42	For whom did this person work? *If now on active duty in the Armed Forces, mark (X) this box ☐* *and print the branch of the Armed Forces.* Name of company, business, or other employer	Industry
43	What kind of business or industry was this? *Describe the activity at the location where employed. (For example: hospital, newspaper publishing, mail order house, auto engine manufacturing, bank)*	
44	Is this mainly–*Mark (X) ONE box.* ☐ manufacturing? ☐ wholesale trade? ☐ retail trade? ☐ other (agriculture, construction, service, government, etc.)?	
45	What kind of work was this person doing? *(For example: registered nurse, personnel manager, supervisor of order department, secretary, accountant)*	Occupation
46	What were this person's most important activities or duties? *(For example: patient care, directing hiring policies, supervising order clerks, typing and filing, reconciling financial records)*	

For the occupation questions, responses such as "day care director" are reported in SOC 11-9030 Education Administrators. Census procedures also use industry information in assigning occupation codes. For example, a response of "director" where the industry Child Day Care Services was assigned would be reported in SOC 11-9030 Education Administrators.

Table B-25 summarizes where workers will be found in the household data by ECCE component. Note that for FCC proprietors, those in incorporated businesses will be found in the same categories as preschool directors in center-based programs: they are either wage and salary workers or self-employed (unincorporated) proprietors in the Child Day Care Services industry, in the occupation the Census occupational equivalent of 11-9030 Education Administrators. Similarly, FCC employees other than proprietors cannot be identified separately from wage and salary workers in center-based programs in the same occupation.

The upshot of this discussion is that, in Census household survey data, identifying formal FCC home-based center proprietors and workers requires cross-tabulating the data by class of worker, industry, and occupation. Identifying FFN caregivers requires a similar cross-tabulation. Cross-tabulations may be produced using the Public Use Microdata Sample (PUMS) files or by the Census Bureau from the full microdata set. Even this type of tabulation likely will include some child care service business owners who operate non-residential-based care services. However, this would be the closest proxy from household data for child care providers who operate out of their residences. Note that the Private Households industry can include only wage and salary workers, and no self-employed workers.

8. *The Current Population Survey does not provide statistically reliable data for small domains because of the limited sample size.*

Some analyses of CPS data in ECCE research examine information at fine levels of detail.[24] Given the CPS sample size, relative standard errors (sampling error) on such data are likely high.

The Census Bureau began publishing data from the ACS with data for 2005. The ACS has a much larger sample and is designed to provide detailed information at various levels of geography for a set of data items similar to or identical to those found in the CPS. The disadvantage of the ACS compared to the CPS is that it is a relatively new survey and thus does not provide a long time series. Also, the ACS is not available

---

[24] For example, Herzenberg et al. (2005). *Losing Ground in Early Childhood Education: Declining Workforce Qualifications in an Expanding Industry, 1979-2004* used CPS data to identify home-based providers in California by highest level of education.

TABLE B-25 Locating Workers in Household Survey Data by ECCE Component

Data Item	Center-Based		School-Based	Family Child Care (FCC) Home-Based Services		Family, Friend, and Neighbor (FFN) Caregivers
	Proprietors	Employees	Employees	Proprietors	Employees	
Class of worker						
Wage and salary worker	Proprietors of incorporated businesses	✓	✓	Proprietors of incorporated businesses	✓	✓
Self-employed worker, not incorporated	Proprietors of unincorporated businesses			Proprietors of unincorporated businesses		✓
Industry	624410 Child day care services	624410 Child day care services	611110 Elementary and secondary schools	624410 Child day care services	624410 Child day care services	624410 Child day care services 814110 Private Households
Occupation	11-9030 Education administrators	11-9030 Education administrators 25-2010 Preschool and kindergarten teachers 25-2050 Special education teachers 39-9011 Child Care workers Other occupations	11-9030 Education administrators 25-2010 Preschool and kindergarten teachers 25-2050 Special education teachers 39-9011 Child Care workers Other occupations	11-9030 Education administrators	39-9011 Child Care workers Other occupations	39-9011 Child Care workers

as quickly as the CPS relative to its reference date, and for some levels of detail, the 3-year or 5-year datasets must be used instead of 1-year data.

Data Currently Available from Department of Labor and Census Bureau Sources

This section provides information about data sources produced by the Department of Labor and the Census Bureau from establishment and household surveys that are relevant to ECCE workforce analysis. Table B-26 lists the data sources reviewed. In the tables that follow, for each data source, certain metadata are identified, followed by a brief assessment of the advantages and limitations of the data source for ECCE purposes.

TABLE B-26 BLS and Census Bureau Data Sources Reviewed

Source	Agency	Type	Description
American Community Survey (ACS)	Census	Household survey	Replaced decennial Census long form. More robust sample size than the CPS allows more data on demographics and wages by occupation, and other characteristics. Includes a question on health insurance coverage
American Time Use Survey (ATUS)	BLS	Household survey	Annual data on the amount of time people spend doing various activities, such as paid work, child care, volunteering, and socializing
Current Employment Statistics (CES)	BLS	Establishment survey	Monthly and annual industry time series on employment, hours, and wages
Current Population Survey (CPS)	BLS/Census	Household survey	Current overall trends in labor force participation, employment and unemployment, and demographics and wages by occupation and industry. Sample size limits demographic and other characteristics detail by occupation and industry
Employment Projections	BLS	Projections	Long-term employment projections by industry and occupation. Career information published in the Occupational Outlook Handbook
National Compensation Survey (NCS)	BLS	Establishment survey	Data on wages and benefits by occupation
Occupational Employment Statistics (OES)	BLS	Establishment survey	Occupational employment and wages, and industry staffing patterns
Occupational Information Network (O*NET)	ETA	Establishment survey of incumbent workers Subject Matter Experts	Comprehensive occupational descriptions and data in the form of rating scales on knowledge, skills, abilities, tasks, and other measures

continued

TABLE B-26 Continued

Source	Agency	Type	Description
Quarterly Census of Employment and Wages (QCEW)	BLS	Establishment administrative data	Monthly, quarterly, and annual data on employment by detailed industry; quarterly and annual data on total payroll and payroll per employee
Survey of Occupational Injuries and Illnesses (SOII)	BLS	Establishment survey	Annual information on the rate, number and severity of work-related non-fatal injuries and illnesses, and how these statistics vary by incident, industry, geography, occupation, and other characteristics

AMERICAN COMMUNITY SURVEY (ACS)

Responsible agency	Census Bureau
Where to find it	http://www.census.gov/acs/www/
Type of source	Household survey
Description	A relatively new survey using a series of monthly samples to produce annually updated data for the same small areas (census tracts and block groups) formerly surveyed via the decennial census long-form sample. Initially, 5 years of samples will be required to produce these small-area data. Once 5 years of data are collected, new small-area data will be produced annually. The ACS also provides 3-year and 1-year data products for larger geographic areas.
Periodicity of the data	Annual
Reference period	Annual
Frequency of publication	Annual
Scope	Total population, including people living in both housing units and group quarters
Classifications used and level of detail	Standard Occupational Classification adapted to Census Occupation Codes. For the 2010 SOC, provides 539 detailed occupations, including 4 military occupations North American Industry Classification System adapted to Census Industry Codes
Geographic detail	
National	✓
Region	✓
State	✓
Metropolitan Area	✓
County	✓
City	✓
Urban/suburban/rural	
Other (describe)	✓ Census tracts and block groups (5-year data)

AMERICAN COMMUNITY SURVEY (ACS) continued

Data elements produced that relate to the desired information	1.a Paid workforce (employment) in occupations related to ECCE 1.c Full-time vs. part-time. Provides usual weeks worked, usual hours per week 2.a Distribution of paid workforce (employment) by occupations and industry 2.c Role and responsibility, represented by occupations 3.a Demographic characteristics: age, education, gender, marital status/marital history, race/ethnicity, income, household composition, poverty status, foreign born, language spoken at home and ability to speak English, and other items 3.b Qualifications: educational attainment, school enrollment, field of degree for bachelor's degree 3.d Labor market information: earnings by type (wages and salaries, self-employment); health insurance coverage; usual weekly hours worked; full-time/part-time; journey to work; means of transportation to work; travel time to work 6.a Distribution by urban/rural location 6.b Socioeconomic status of community

Advantages for ECCE purposes:
1. Along with the CPS, the ACS is a comprehensive source of demographic information of workers by occupation, including data on educational attainment, gender, age, race/ethnicity, and other characteristics of workers in the occupations of interest to ECCE.
2. Along with the CPS, the ACS is a source of employment data by occupation for workers in private households.
3. Compared to the CPS, the ACS provides much greater occupational, geographic, and other detail because of the larger sample sizes.
4. Cross-tabulations can be created using the Public Use Microdata Samples (PUMS).

Limitations for ECCE purposes:
1. The ACS is not as timely as the CPS.
2. Limitations of the SOC for identifying ECCE workforce. In addition, the Census Occupational Classification does not provide full SOC detail for preschool teachers or education administrators.
3. Limitations of the NAICS for ECCE purposes.
4. Compared to the OES, occupation by industry information not as detailed or current.

AMERICAN TIME USE SURVEY (ATUS)

Responsible agency	Sponsored by Bureau of Labor Statistics, conducted by Census Bureau
Where to find it	http://www.bls.gov/tus
Type of source	Household survey
Description	Produces estimates of how people spend their time, including time spent doing child care, housework, and volunteering, as well as where and with whom each activity occurred, and whether the activities were done for one's job or business. Demographic information—including sex, race, age, educational attainment, occupation, income, marital status, and the presence of children in the household—also is available for each respondent. Individuals are randomly selected from a subset of households that have completed their eighth and final month of interviews for the Current Population Survey (CPS)
Periodicity of the data	Annual
Reference period	Continuous collection asks one-time respondents about activities starting at 4 a.m. the previous day and ending at 4 a.m. on the interview day.
Frequency of publication	Microdata files published annually; Annual news release
Scope	All residents living in households in the United States that are at least 15 years of age, with the exception of active military personnel and people residing in institutions such as nursing homes and prisons
Classifications used and level of detail	Census 2007 industry classification derived from the NAICS Census 2002 Occupation classification derived from the SOC
Geographic detail	
National	✓
Region	
State	
Metropolitan Area	
County	
City	
Urban/suburban/rural	
Other (describe)	

AMERICAN TIME USE SURVEY (ATUS) (continued)

Data elements produced that relate to the desired information	1.b Unpaid caregivers and 2.a Type of setting. Use ATUS to identify sub-samples of adults who care for their own children and for other people's children, but who do not list child care as their occupation.
	Use ATUS to distinguish time spent doing primary from secondary care by both parents and other caregivers to adjust other data on parent-reported hours in parental or FFN care to reflect only primary caregiving hours.
	For parental and FFN caregivers, use ATUS for estimating the value of the wages foregone while they are caring for young children.

Advantages for ECCE purposes:
1.   Time use data provide a proxy for more direct measures of FFN care and for estimating costs of care outside formal settings.

Limitations for ECCE purposes:
1.   Not a direct measure of employment or wages.

CURRENT EMPLOYMENT STATISTICS (CES)

Responsible agency	Bureau of Labor Statistics
Where to find it	http://www.bls.gov/ces
Type of source	Establishment survey
Description	Produces current detailed industry data on employment, hours, and earnings of workers on nonfarm payrolls
Periodicity of the data	Monthly, Annual
Reference period	Any part of the pay period that includes the 12th day of the month
Frequency of publication	Monthly, Annual
Scope	Excludes proprietors, the unincorporated self-employed, unpaid volunteer or family employees, farm employees, and domestic employees. Salaried officers of corporations are included. Government employment covers only civilian employees; military personnel are excluded.
Classifications used and level of detail	2007 NAICS, Industry-specific estimates for NAICS sectors, 3-digit, 4-digit, and 5-digit
Geographic detail	
National	✓
Region	✓
State	✓
Metropolitan Area	✓ MSA ✓ MSA divisions

County
   City
   Urban/suburban/rural
   Other (describe)	

Data elements produced that relate to the desired information	1.a Paid workforce. Monthly and annual estimates for industries relevant to ECCE, including employment, average weekly hours, average hourly earnings for both total and production and nonsupervisory workers. Number of women employees

Advantages for ECCE purposes:
1. The CES is very timely.
2. Provides current employment trends for ECCE industries at the state and MSA levels, although availability may vary.

Limitations for ECCE purposes:
1. Limitations of the NAICS for identifying ECCE establishments.
2. Excludes wage and salary workers in private households.
3. Does not include self-employed workers.
4. Does not provide occupational data.
5. Does not provide information on worker demographics (except for gender), qualifications, or preparation.

CURRENT POPULATION SURVEY (CPS)

Responsible agency	Joint program of the Bureau of Labor Statistics and the Census Bureau
Where to find it	http://www.census.gov/cps/
Type of source	Household survey
Description	Monthly survey of about 60,000 households. Primary source of data on the labor force characteristics of the U.S. population, as well as income and poverty status
Periodicity of the data	Monthly, Annual
Reference period	Generally the week including the 12th of the month
Frequency of publication	Monthly, Quarterly, Annual
Scope	Civilian noninstitutional population. Respondents are interviewed to obtain information about the employment status of each member of the household 15 years of age and older. However, published data focus on those ages 16 and over.
Classifications used and level of detail	Standard Occupational Classification adapted to Census Occupation Codes. For the 2010 SOC, provides 539 detailed occupations. The NAICS adapted to Census Industry Codes.
Geographic detail	
National	✓ The sample provides labor force characteristics for the nation and serves as part of model-based estimates for individual states and other geographic areas.
Region	Some regional data available
State	Some state data available
Metropolitan Area	
County	
City	
Urban/suburban/rural	
Other (describe)	

CURRENT POPULATION SURVEY (CPS) (continued)

Data elements produced that relate to the desired information	1.a Paid workforce (employment) in occupations related to ECCE
	1.c Full-time vs. part-time. Provides usual weeks worked, usual hours per week
	2.c Role and responsibility, represented by occupations
	3.a Demographic characteristics: age, education, gender, marital status, race/ethnicity, income, foreign born, and other items
	3.b Qualifications: educational attainment, school enrollment
	3.d Labor market information: usual weekly earnings by type (for wage and salary workers); health insurance coverage; hours worked; at work part-time for economic reasons; multiple job-holding

Advantages for ECCE purposes:
1. Along with the ACS, the CPS is a comprehensive source of demographic information of workers by occupation, including data on educational attainment, gender, age, race/ethnicity, and other characteristics.
2. Along with the ACS, the CPS is a source of employment data by occupation for workers in private households.
3. The CPS is very timely.
4. Cross-tabulations can be created using the Public Use Microdata Samples (PUMS). However, some results may be unreliable because of small sample size.

Limitations for ECCE purposes:
1. Compared to the ACS, the CPS provides much less occupational, geographic, and other detail because of the smaller sample size.
2. Limitations of the SOC for identifying ECCE workforce. In addition, the Census Occupational Classification does not provide full SOC detail for preschool teachers or education administrators.

NOTE: BLS: Bureau of Labor Statistics; ETA: Employment and Training Administration.

EMPLOYMENT PROJECTIONS (EP) PROGRAM

Responsible agency	Bureau of Labor Statistics
Where to find it	http://www.bls.gov/emp/
Type of source	Combines estimates from establishment and household surveys
Description	10-year projections, by industry and occupation, developed primarily using data from the OES, CES, and CPS
Periodicity of the data	New projections produced every two years.
Reference period	2008-2018
Frequency of publication	Every 2 years
Scope	All employed workers are included in total employment as a count of jobs, all classes of worker
Classifications used and level of detail	SOC 2000 6-digit detailed occupations. Excludes military occupations (SOC Major Group 55) NAICS 2007 industry-specific estimates at 4-digit level, except Educational Services at 3-digit level. Selected 5-digit industry levels
Geographic detail	
National	✓
Region	
State	State and area projections produced by state agencies, not part of BLS program. See http://www.projectionscentral.com
Metropolitan Area	
County	
City	
Urban/suburban/rural	
Other (describe)	
Data elements produced that relate to the desired information	1.a Paid workforce. Long-term projections of demand by occupation and industry

Advantages for ECCE purposes:
1. Provides long-term projections of employment and job openings for occupations and employment by industry.
2. Career information products are available based on the employment projections analysis.

Limitations for ECCE purposes:
1. Limitations of the SOC for identifying ECCE workforce.
2. Limitations of the NAICS for ECCE purposes.

NATIONAL COMPENSATION SURVEY (NCS)

Responsible agency	Bureau of Labor Statistics
Where to find it	http://www.bls.gov/ncs/
Type of source	Establishment survey
Description	Provides comprehensive measures of occupational wages by detailed occupation. Employment cost trends; and benefit incidence and detailed plan provisions, by occupational grouping
Periodicity of the data	Continuous
Reference period	Varies. Data published in the 2009 national bulletin for occupational earnings were compiled from data collected between December 2008 and January 2010. The average reference period is July 2009
Frequency of publication	Occupational pay and benefits incidence—Annual Employment costs—Monthly
Scope	Includes non-farm private, state government, and local government. Excludes federal, agricultural, and household workers, and self-employed workers
Classifications used and level of detail	Occupational pay—2000 SOC, 6-digit detailed occupations. Excludes military occupations (SOC major group 55) Employment cost trends; and benefit incidence and detailed plan provisions, by occupational grouping
Geographic detail	
National	✓
Region	✓
State	✓
Metropolitan Area	✓ Selected MSAs
County	
City	
Urban/suburban/rural	
Other (describe)	✓ Selected Micropolitan areas
Data elements produced that relate to the desired information	3.d Labor market information: benefits; wages by full-time/part-time, and by union status

Advantages for ECCE purposes:
1. Provides information on benefits by occupation, and relative wages by full-time/part-time and union/nonunion status.

Limitations for ECCE purposes:
1. Occupational and geographic detail limited by small sample sizes.
2. Limitations of the SOC for identifying ECCE workforce.
3. Limitations of the NAICS for ECCE purposes.
4. Excludes self-employed workers.
5. Excludes private households.

OCCUPATIONAL EMPLOYMENT STATISTICS (OES) PROGRAM

Responsible agency	Bureau of Labor Statistics
Where to find it	http://www.bls.gov/oes
Type of source	Establishment survey
Description	Produces employment and wage estimates for over 800 occupations, with breakouts by industry
Periodicity of the data	Annual
Reference period	May of reference year
Frequency of publication	Annual
Scope	Wage and salary employment in all industries except private households and most agriculture industries
Classifications used and level of detail	Standard Occupational Classification, 6-digit detailed occupations. Excludes military occupations (SOC Major Group 23) The NAICS, industry-specific estimates for NAICS sectors, 3-digit, 4-digit, and selected 5-digit industry levels.
Geographic detail	
National	✓
Region	
State	✓
Metropolitan Area	✓ MSA ✓ MSA Divisions
County	
City	
Urban/suburban/rural	
Other (describe)	Balance of state areas composed of non-metropolitan geography in each state

OCCUPATIONAL EMPLOYMENT STATISTICS (OES) PROGRAM (continued)

Data elements produced that relate to the desired information	1.a Paid workforce (employment) in detailed SOC occupations related to ECCE
	2.a Distribution of paid workforce (employment) in occupations related to ECCE by industry, including especially NAICS 611110 Elementary and Secondary Schools, and 624410 Child Day Care Services
	2.c Role and responsibility, represented by occupations
	3.d Compensation, specifically hourly wages in occupations related to ECCE, total by geographic area, and nationally by industry
	5.a Distribution of staffing by roles, represented by occupations, within industries
	6.a Distribution by urban/rural location. OES data can be tabulated to urban/rural using the MSA and balance of state (non-metropolitan) area data

Advantages for ECCE purposes:
1. Comprehensive source of employment and wage information by occupation for wage and salary workers.
2. Data available by occupation by industry, indicating variations in wages by industry as well as occupational distribution (staffing pattern) of employment in specific industries.
3. Large sample size results in data in significant occupational, industry, and geographic detail.

Limitations for ECCE purposes:
1. Limitations of the SOC for identifying ECCE workforce.
2. Limitations of the NAICS for identifying ECCE establishments.
3. Excludes wage and salary workers in private households.
4. Does not provide information on worker demographics, qualifications, or preparation.

OCCUPATIONAL INFORMATION NETWORK (O*NET)

Responsible agency	Employment and Training Administration, U.S. Department of Labor
Where to find it	http://www.onetonline.org/ (provides O*NET data access, provides documentation, data downloads, and other information)
Type of source	Establishment survey (two-stage survey to obtain sample of job incumbents within sampled establishments) Subject matter experts
Description	Provides comprehensive occupational descriptions and data in the form of several hundred rating scales on knowledge, skills, abilities, tasks, and other measures. The O*NET Content Model was developed using research on job and organizational analysis and includes job-oriented descriptors and worker-oriented descriptors.
Periodicity of the data	Updates to database added approximately annual as data from recent collections are incorporated
Reference period	Not applicable
Frequency of publication	Approximately annually
Scope	Wage and salary employment in all industries except private households and most agriculture industries
Classifications used and level of detail	SOC, 6-digit detailed occupations with additional detail for some occupations. Excludes military occupations (SOC Major Group 55)

Geographic detail
   National
   Region
   State
   Metropolitan Area
   County
   City
   Urban/suburban/rural
   Other (describe)
	✓

OCCUPATIONAL INFORMATION NETWORK (O*NET) (continued)

Data elements produced that relate to the desired information	No specific data elements. However, O*NET information can be useful in understanding the child care workforce in terms of the characteristics in the O*NET Content Model: Worker Characteristics (Abilities, Interests, Work Styles, Work Values) Worker Requirements (Skills, Knowledge, Education) Experience Requirements (Experience and Training, Basic and Cross-functional Skills Entry Requirements, Licensing) Occupational Requirements (Generalized and Detailed Work Activities, Organizational and Work Context) Occupation-specific Information (Tasks, Tools and Technology)

Advantages for ECCE purposes:
1. Comprehensive source of information on tasks performed, skills, abilities, and other measures.

Limitations for ECCE purposes:
1. Limitations of the SOC for identifying ECCE workforce.
2. No data collected from wage and salary workers in private households.

QUARTERLY CENSUS OF EMPLOYMENT AND WAGES (QCEW)

Responsible agency	Bureau of Labor Statistics
Where to find it	http://www.bls.gov/cew
Type of source	Administrative
Description	Produces monthly, quarterly, and annual data on employment and wages. Quarterly and annual data on total payroll and payroll per employee. First quarter data on establishment size class
Periodicity of the data	Monthly, quarterly, and annual
Reference period	Any part of the pay period that includes the 12th day of the month
Frequency of publication	Quarterly
Scope	The QCEW program derives its data from quarterly tax reports submitted to State Employment Security Agencies by more than 8 million employers subject to state unemployment insurance (UI) laws and from federal agencies subject to the Unemployment Compensation for Federal Employees (UCFE) program. The QCEW program has data on nonagricultural industries, along with partial information on agricultural industries and employees in private households. For the first quarter of each year, data are tabulated by establishment size class. The size category of each establishment is determined by the March employment level. These size class data are available at the national level by NAICS industry, and at the state level by NAICS sector.
Classifications used and level of detail	2007 NAICS, Industry-specific estimates for NAICS sectors, 3-digit, 4-digit, and 5-digit
Geographic detail	
National	✓
Region	✓
State	✓
Metropolitan Area	✓ Consolidated Metropolitan Statistical Areas ✓ Metropolitan Statistical Areas
County	✓
City	
Urban/suburban/rural	
Other (describe)	Individual establishment records are geo-coded.
Data elements produced that relate to the desired information	1.a Paid workforce. Monthly and annual estimates for industries relevant to ECCE, including employment, number of establishments, total payroll, and payroll per employee

QUARTERLY CENSUS OF EMPLOYMENT AND WAGES (QCEW) (continued)

Advantages for ECCE purposes:

1. Provides data on employment, number of establishments, total payroll, and payroll per employee for ECCE industries at full NAICS and geographic detail, except where data subject to protection of confidentiality.
2. Includes wage and salary workers in private households.

Limitations for ECCE purposes:

1. Compared to CES, QCEW is much less timely.
2. Limitations of the NAICS for identifying ECCE establishments.
3. Excludes employment not subject to unemployment insurance coverage, which may affect inclusion domestic workers in private households.
4. Does not include self-employed workers.
5. Does not provide occupational data.
6. Does not provide information on worker demographics (except for gender), qualifications, or preparation.

SURVEY OF OCCUPATIONAL INJURIES AND ILLNESSES (SOII)

Responsible agency	Bureau of Labor Statistics
Where to find it	http://www.bls.gov/iif/home.htm
Type of source	Establishment survey
Description	Provides annual information on the rate, number, and severity of work-related non-fatal injuries and illnesses, and how these statistics vary by incident, industry, geography, occupation, and other characteristics
Periodicity of the data	Annual
Reference period	Calendar year
Frequency of publication	Annual
Scope	Employers having 11 employees or more in agricultural production, all employers in all other private industries and state and local government. Excludes self-employed persons and workers in private households (NAICS 814), the U.S. Postal Service (NAICS 491), and the federal government
Classifications used and level of detail	SOC 2000 6-digit detailed occupations. Does not include SOC residuals or military occupations (SOC major group 55) NAICS 2007 publishable data include 3-digit Educational Services, 4-digit Child Day Care Services
Geographic detail	
National	✓
Region	
State	44 participating states, the District of Columbia, and territories (for 2009)
Metropolitan Area	
County	
City	
Urban/suburban/rural	
Other (describe)	
Data elements produced that relate to the desired information	3.d Labor market information: number and rate of illnesses and injuries by occupation and industry

Advantages for ECCE purposes:
1. Source of injury and illness information for occupations and industries of interest to ECCE.

Limitations for ECCE purposes:
1. Some states not participating, although national data include samples from all states.
2. Excludes self-employed workers.
3. Excludes private households, U.S. Postal Services, and federal workers.
4. Limitations of the SOC for identifying ECCE workforce.
5. Limitations of the NAICS for ECCE purposes.